HEALTH ASPECTS OF AGING

HEALTH ASPECTS OF AGING

The Experience of Growing Old

By

GARI LESNOFF-CARAVAGLIA, PH.D.

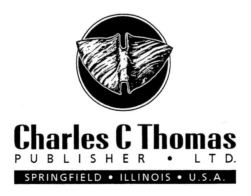

Charles C Thomas
PUBLISHER • LTD.
SPRINGFIELD • ILLINOIS • U.S.A.

Published and Distributed Throughout the World by

CHARLES C THOMAS • PUBLISHER, LTD.
2600 South First Street
Springfield, Illinois 62704

©2000 by CHARLES C THOMAS • PUBLISHER, LTD.

ISBN 0-398-07011-3 (cloth)
ISBN 0-398-07012-1 (paper)

Library of Congress Catalog Card Number: 99-044461

With THOMAS BOOKS *careful attention is given to all details of manufacturing
and design. It is the Publisher's desire to present books that are satisfactory as to their
physical qualities and artistic possibilities and appropriate for their particular use.*
THOMAS BOOKS *will be true to those laws of quality that assure a good name
and good will.*

Printed in the United States of America
CR-R-3

Library of Congress Cataloging-in-Publication Data

Lesnoff-Caravaglia, Gari.
    Health aspects of aging : the experience of growing old
    Gari Lesnoff-Caravalglia.
        p. cm.
    Includes bibliographical references and index.
    ISBN 0-398-07011-3 (cloth) ISBN 0-398-07012-1 (paper)
        1. Aging. 2.Aged--Health and Hygiene. I. Title.
    [DNLM: 1. Aging--physiology. 2. Health Services for the Aged.
WT 31 L637h 2000]
QP86 .L47 2000
613'.0438--dc21   99-044461

PREFACE

The growing presence of large numbers of persons aged 65 and older worldwide no longer calls forth surprise nor alarm, and has permitted a more ordered view of human existence. This recent orientation has also led to a life span perspective, with late life taking on its proper dimension within such ordering, whilst the problem approach to aging has been replaced by a problem-solving approach.

Such a problem-solving approach has not only allowed for the perception of late life as a normal progression but has also encouraged the development of intervention and prevention strategies to offset debilities due to such causes as the aging of the human organism, the onslaught of disease, an incongruous environment, or altered social states. The experience of life into very advanced old age continues to unmask negative stereotypes and to foster its accommodation into the normal patterning of human existence.

The aim of science and medicine is less to lengthen life and more to reduce the number of years that people spend diseased or disabled. Healthy aging is clearly possible, and those who are rich, well-educated, do not smoke, and are physically active do seem to be experiencing what has been termed a "compression of morbidity" in that their extra years of life are largely healthy.

Although old age is associated with disease, it does not cause it. All major adult diseases tend to be much more common in old age than in early adult life due to a number of factors, including that of long life. Much of the misdiagnosis and overlooking of symptoms in the elderly is due to negative stereotyping and repugnance toward the older body. Studies indicate that physicians rarely examine the breasts of older women even when there are strong clinical indications for doing so.

The presence of increasing numbers of older persons in the population can lead to challenges and creative responses to a new and dynamic change in the demography. Such alterations in the composition of the population, if not adequately subsumed and prepared for, can also lead to chaos. Aging affects everything from cells, physiological systems, clinical medicine, society, economics, to ethics. Aging has become an important issue because of dramatic changes in life expectancy. In developed countries those aged over 80 are the fastest-growing section of the population. In the developing world, 60 percent of the people are over 60, and it will rise to 80 percent by the middle of the next century. The number of older persons will outnumber children in the near future. Society is not well prepared for the fall in birth rates and the rise in life expectancy.

The disease burden associated with increased life expectations has massive implications for health policy. A multidisciplinary approach is essential for the understanding of aging and for effective management of chronic disease. The distinction between health and social care will very likely diminish in the future as persons continue to live to advanced ages.

The chapters in this volume address these issues from the perspectives of diverse disciplines and professional standpoints. Since biological changes are key issues, the aging process is largely described from the perspective of biological changes related to age and to particular dysfunctions. The environmental features and the potential introduction of technological interventions are interspersed within chapters, as well as finding primary focus in particular chapters.

Gari Lesnoff-Caravaglia

CONTENTS

HEALTH ASPECTS OF AGING

Chapter 1

HEALTH ASPECTS OF AGING:
AN INTRODUCTION

The world has assumed a new look or new dimension due to two primary changes. One is the result of the increasing number of older persons found throughout the world, and the second is the product of the fact that technological advances have radically altered daily existence. Such changes reflect both potential positive and negative aspects as they affect individuals, society, the notion of community, life-styles, opportunities and responsibilities. In the United States, the nation's older population will more than double by the year 2050. That population will be more racially and ethnically diverse than ever before.

At the turn of the century, life expectancy was approximately 49, and the median age was 22.9. Today, people live a quarter of a century longer with the life expectancy for women now reaching 83 and for men 78. The number of years persons lived as postparental years in 1940 was 17 years; it is currently 33 years. Married women can expect to live 20 to 30 years with a spouse, whereas in 1800, the expectation was 12 years. Sixty-eight percent of all women are widows at 75. Women, also, make up two-thirds of the population over the age of 75.

Older persons continue to play significant roles in all areas of life. Many continue to perform in the workplace, at home, and in professional spheres. Many persons, although advanced in age, do not regard themselves as "old." Older persons are also found in the criminal world, as well as in the higher estates of life. For example, a woman aged 80 was recently apprehended at an international airport smuggling vast quantities of cocaine hidden under her girdle. She is the oldest suspected drug smuggler to be arrested by British customs.

As the population continues to age, older persons are found to be involved in all aspects of life—both the positive and the negative.

Understanding Aging

Although it is recognized that biological changes are inevitable as part of the aging process, it is not clear why such changes occur. The process of aging is poorly understood. An ancient belief held that there was a magic elixir or potion that could halt aging or retard its progress. The explorer Ponce de Leon was sent to the New World by Queen Isabella of Spain to find the fountain of youth. She was worried that her husband, King Ferdinand, who was reported to be several years her junior, would lose interest in her as she grew older. Ponce de Leon did not find the fountain of youth, but he discovered Florida. The Florida that, curiously enough, became the haven of the elderly of today.

Contemporary theories of aging cannot account for why it is that people age. One theory, the wear and tear theory, maintains that the body simply wears out over time. Other theories deal with the changes within the cells themselves, while still others state that aging is programmed, and that the aging process is regulated by an aging clock located in the hypothalamus. The gene theory maintains that there are certain genes which contribute to bodily dysfunctions, and that these genes appear to become activated as persons grow older. Further, there is the cellular garbage theory that claims that there are certain deposits (such as lipofuscin) that accumulate in cells to create dysfunctions that lead to aging and, ultimately, death.

The autoimmune theory is very likely the theory that should receive greater attention. According to this theory, the immune system gradually breaks down, and, thus, permits certain diseases to be activated in old age or to cause diseases of long maturation to manifest themselves in old age. This results from the fact that the immune system in older persons appears to function less efficiently.

No theory adequately explains why people age, or how they age. Some hypotheses promulgated to help retard the aging process have included: lowering the caloric intake, sleeping in colder environments, or developing special diets. The ideal is to keep people young for as long as possible, and to avoid old age altogether.

Aging occurs within the body at the cellular level, as well as outwardly. Yet it is the outward signs that are referred to when commonly describing aging. The graying of the hair, wrinkled skin, loss of hair, stooped posture, or other alterations in appearance. In some older persons, the posture is so bent that the person appears to be facing the ground. There is an old saying that the grave is already beckoning this person.

Chronological Age

Chronological age refers to the number of years a person has lived or an individual's birthday age. There is also the term physiological age. This is the physical age of the person. An individual may be 90 years old, but have the health status that is equivalent to a 50-year-old. A person at age 60 suffering from a heart ailment may have a heart that can be equated to that of an 80-year-old. Even within one individual, organs age at different rates. A person's kidneys may be one age, the heart another, and the liver still another.

One overarching change that is linked to the aging of an individual is the fact that he or she responds less well to stress. More time is required to recover from stress. There is also an inherent vulnerability that accompanies the aging process. Persons who appear hale and hearty prior to a stressful event, such as experiencing a fall, may have great difficulty, physically and psychologically, in overcoming resultant trauma or stress.

Increased Longevity

Advances in medical knowledge, combined with better dietary and sanitary measures, have led to an increase in life expectancy. An increase in the number of elderly people is accompanied by a greater incidence of the health disorders of the aged.

The aging of the population is a universal change, and has kindled increased interest in the study of population changes or demography. Since the 1880s there has been a gradual increase in life expectancy.

Longevity refers to the length of life. Demographers study the statistical characteristics of populations throughout the life spans of their members. They provide information about the average (mean) life

Health Aspects of Aging

expectancy, maximum life span, and survivorship curves. Two approaches are used to examine a population on the basis of age. The cross-sectional approach measures the characteristics of existing groups of people and observes how they compare or contrast according to age. The longitudinal approach selects a group of people of the same age and follows changes in their attributes as time passes. The cross-sectional approach has the limitation that each age-based subgroup has had a different biomedical history that may have uniquely influenced the characteristics measured. Following a group throughout its life span (longitudinal) is expensive, and, at each successive stage of study, the survivors are unique.

A conspicuous feature of an aged population is the range, or variability, of function seen in any given age group. An individual, age 70, who is near death and has many systems failing to maintain homeostasis, provides a notable contrast with those of the same age and in good health who may expect to live another 10 to 30 years. This variability is not trivial to the understanding of age changes. It is not surprising, for example, that older persons have nutritional needs and metabolic characteristics that are different and more limiting than those of their youth. If there is no particular value to the species in these functions lasting in optimal form beyond the reproductive period of life, then some may deteriorate as aging occurs, while others randomly persist. Gerontologists, who study all aspects of aging, and geriatricians, the biomedical group interested in the health of the aged, must look at the aged as a population in which some of the physiological characteristics of the young continue, but in which other characteristics become altered in an irregular way and need new understanding.

The study of aging must be multidisciplinary, drawing substantially from fields of study such as sociology, psychology, biology, genetics, and biochemistry. Physiology remains central in considering the mechanisms of the body and the processes by which they are carried out.

Life Expectancy and Life Span

Life expectancy varies and changes, and there has been a gradual increase over time, since approximately the middle 1850s. At the turn of the century, if an individual had reached the age of 50, this individual was considered to be old. People who reached the age of 50 were regarded in the same light as are people today who are 125. They were considered to be the very old persons in the society.

People did not live as long in earlier times. There were a number of reasons to account for their shorter lives. The standard of living was lower, there were more environmental dangers, and women died in childbirth more often. Currently, health concerns have been more successfully resolved due, in part, to the presence of advanced technologies allowing people to experience new health care interventions. Health care intervention has changed, along with the educational levels of the population.

Some persons currently in their eighties and nineties did not progress beyond the sixth grade. It was unusual in their age cohort for an individual to have graduated from high school. It was not until after World War II that many people who were not affluent had the opportunity to attend institutions of higher learning. This was largely due to the G.I. Bill which permitted people who had served in the armed services an opportunity to advance their educations. With the expansion of educational opportunities, people were more sophisticated with respect to caring for their health and as to their expectations with regard to health and social services. They have also become aware of the relationship between political astuteness and the ability to seek services through active political participation. People increasingly take an entrepreneurial attitude toward their own health care and needs and want to participate in the decision-making process that intimately affects them. This attitude has brought about changes in the doctor/patient relationship. People have also become aware of the relationship between more healthful life-styles, better health care, and personal longevity. They also realize that better education, better jobs, and higher incomes all lead to increases in life expectancy.

Better sanitary systems, the control of pests, improved plumbing, have all led to further increases in life expectancy. This has led to the absence of plagues such as the bubonic plague or the black plague that used to obliterate large sections of the world. Entire cities would disappear from the face of the earth.

There are, also, gender differences with respect to life expectancy. In most industrialized nations, women live longer than do men. This is due in part to the fact that men are exposed to a greater number of hazards related to their work environments and often lead life-styles that include the abuse of alcohol and tobacco. All of these factors significantly reduce life expectancy.

Life expectancy for females is approximately 6 to 10 years greater than it is for males. Environmental factors for women are different from those of men. Men are more prone to experience industrial accidents, are more often exposed to toxic substances, are involved in greater numbers in automobile accidents, are involved in greater numbers of suicidal and homicidal deaths, and are more likely to engage in unhealthful life-styles. As a result, in most industrialized societies, the life expectancy for women exceeds that of men.

Some population groups experience shorter life expectancies. Life-style can also militate against long life. For example, Native Americans have very short life expectancies compared to White Americans due, in part, to poor nutrition, poor health facilities, and abuse of alcohol and tobacco. The life expectancy for a male Native American is approximately 45 years of age. The life expectancy for the average White American male is approximately 78 years of age.

Formerly, it was common for persons to enter custodial care settings, such as nursing homes, when they were about 62 years of age. It is more common for persons to enter nursing homes at an age closer to 90; the average age is 86.

Mandatory retirement age for many years was placed at 65 years of age. Persons had to leave their positions, their jobs, and their professional associations. Mandatory retirement has been effectively abolished, primarily because it became meaningless. People became healthier and were able to continue in their work activities. Concomitantly, there was a change in demography, resulting in changes within the population structure. There was no longer the presence of large groups of young people. The knowledge and expertise of older workers was needed and led to the abandonment of mandatory retirement to allow persons to remain longer in the workplace.

The establishment of age 65 as a retirement age was an arbitrary one. It was not based on biological or psychological aging, or serious studies of the detriments of maintaining the older worker. Age 65 had been established in Germany by Bismarck who determined that persons who had worked long and hard to establish the current society should be rewarded by an acknowledgement of this contribution to the welfare of the state by a pension plan. The plan was to go into effect when persons reached the age of 65. He picked that age because in that time period few people lived long enough to reach this age, and, consequently, since the number of persons who could claim such pension benefits would be small, the burden on state coffers would be light. No one, of course, could predict that life expectancy would increase dramatically, and that, in the scheme of things, people in the future who reached age 65 would not be considered old at all.

Nonetheless, age 65 was seized upon by the rest of the world as a chronological marker with respect to age. After age 65, people were to be retired from work and were, in general, to be regarded as the older portion of the population. Age 65 thus took on a negative connotation, and, since much attention is paid to individuals' ages, to say one was 65 was tantamount to admitting to being old and non-productive. Lying about one's age probably increased in momentum due to the negative stereotyping of older individuals. There was the growth of ageism, a negative way of regarding older persons much as is sexism or racism. A negative climate was developed which included sayings such as: "You can't teach an old dog new tricks."

In the United States, the Social Security Act was instituted in the early 1930s to principally assist persons with little or no income to subsist in old age. The intention originally was to provide some assistance, but not to provide totally for an individual's needs. This notion changed over the years, and many people do, in fact, have only Social Security benefits to support them in their old age.

There is nothing biologically, sociologically, or psychologically, that determined that age 65 was an appropriate age to limit persons' work activity. Older women, in particular, suffered from the negative stereotyping associated with growing older. Women not only suffered from ageism, but, if they belonged to a minority group, they suffered racism, and, being women, they also faced sexism. Such prejudice is heightened by the fact that 50 percent of the older women, as compared to older men, live below the poverty level.

Life span, on the other hand, is species determined. There are mice that live six months and insects that live only hours. The average life span for the cat is approximately 25 years, the dog 30 years, the horse 30 years, some turtles 200 years, and some birds 100 years. The life span for the human species for some time had been considered as 100 years, but the figure now accepted is 125 years.

Everything ages. Not only human beings, but material things as well. Wood, furniture, buildings, cities, sections of cities, trees, ore deep in the ground, all age. Everything goes through the aging process. This is true of human beings as well. At the time of conception, the individual begins the process of aging. People age over time, and their aging is manifest in their appearance, interests, and life experiences. Changes are more rapid at certain periods of life, such as infancy, but changes continue to occur, perhaps more subtly in later stages of development. Some changes are viewed with joy and anticipated, others at other stages of life appear depressing, and there may be the wish to conceal or hide such changes.

In the western world, most cultures are future time oriented. People plan their lives in terms of future expected events and pay little heed to the past or its influence. Such future time orientation created a problem for the older population. Such an emphasis upon the future diminished the importance of past events and lives already lived. When individuals reached 65, they felt apprehensive about their lives, depressed that there was little to look forward to as they had been asked to retire from their jobs. Death was the only future life event. The denial of aging and death resulted from an overly stressed future time orientation. Life was not perceived as a progression from birth to death, but rather birth to retirement. Those who continued to live beyond age 65 were hard-pressed to give life meaning. Some engaged in reminiscence, some became ill, while others fought against the established norms which gave rise to groups such as the Gray Panthers.

Reminiscence was heralded as a positive life review. Such a hanging on to significant events of the past was probably the only way older persons had to hold on to their personal integrity, and was rather more symptomatic of the unsympathetic climate in which aging was experienced rather than a healthy looking back at one's life and trying to provide it with meaning and coherence. As a result, many older persons were guilty of repeatedly recounting past experiences which they felt were significant and only succeeded in boring relatives. For example, one grandmother repeatedly related in great detail how she came to America in the hold of a ship, barefoot and alone. The reason for such repetition is that the older person does not have new experiences, or interesting current events to relate, and thus to appear interesting, focuses on past dramatic episodes. This also partially explains the sick role played by older persons to gain attention of children. The sick role is acceptable, whereas the role of older person is fraught with ambiguity.

The chronological age of 65 as the hallmark of aging also meant that older persons were categorically regarded as ill or prone to soon become so, and health care providers were reluctant to spend time on older patients. They were regarded as already doomed, and intervention was seen as futile. The ignoring of health care needs of older persons still finds its reverberation today in the lack of support for research on the diseases which primarily affect the elderly. This also in part accounts for the lack of adequate mental health care, as well.

A further negative aspect of the emphasis upon chronological age is that aging became associated with death. At the turn of the century, death was more common among children. Family plots in older cemeteries include as many as thirteen children, many of whom lived less than six months. Because of better standards of living and health care, the infant mortality rate has been reduced, and death now occurs more frequently among older persons. Although with increases in life expectancy, older persons live longer lives, and the age group 85 and older continues to expand.

Old age, in and of itself, is not a disease. It is not a sickness that gradually overwhelms persons if they live long enough. Rather, aging is a process that occurs over time and is initiated at conception and continues until the organism expires. Aging is experienced at different rates by individuals, and the rate of aging is affected by a wide variety of factors including heredity, life-style, economics, and the environment.

The older client in visiting the physician is often presented with the question: "What do you expect at your age?" Older persons expect answers and diagnoses of their conditions in the same way as do younger individuals.

Older persons are probably more different one from the other, than any other age group. They differ more than do adolescents who certainly have major differences among them. One of the reasons why older persons differ so much from one another is that they have all had differing life experiences. Such differences include their social experience, health history, experience of life events, education, and personal history. When the medical history is taken of an older person, much of this personal equation must be included. This is why geriatrics, the study of the diseases of aging, a medical specialty, must focus on the individual, not just the disease process. Geriatrics was not seriously studied until the end of World War II. Another area of study, gerontology, focuses on the processes of aging from a multidisciplinary perspective. Some hospitals may have a gerontology unit which assists in the evaluation and placement of individuals in long-term care settings.

Religion and Wars

The two important factors that affect society in terms of health care and its provision are religion and wars. Religion has played a significant role in the development of health care and the development of health care institutions. Early hospitals were constructed in the shape of a cross, and the religious concept of caring for others further fostered the presence of religious bodies in health care. The first nurses were monks, and there are many orders of nuns who specialized in nursing care.

Wars helped to spread medical information, and soldiers often returned from distant lands with new knowledge in health care and new interventions. This was particularly true of the crusades which, although a religious war, resulted in bringing significant medical knowledge from the East and North Africa to the European continent. This was a significant avenue for the exchange of information between differing cultures. The American Civil War was also a time for new medical discoveries. Anesthetics, surgery, embalming (preparing dead soldiers to send back to their families) and rehabilitation including prosthetic devices and artificial limbs were all results of treating the injured with greater effectiveness.

World War II revolutionized health care. The MASH units of World War II were largely responsible for the introduction of radical surgeries and treatment modalities into the health care field. Providing care with minimal medical assistance or medications called for extensive innovation. Having to make do with just what was available proved to be a remarkable lesson for many health care units. In emergency situations, they dared the impossible, and often succeeded. This daring spirit is what sparked the burgeoning of advanced health care technologies following World War II.

Increasing Life Expectancy

Life-style is probably a major determinant as to an individual's life expectancy. How one lives one's life will determine its length. The analogy of the machine is a pertinent one. An automobile that is properly maintained, is regularly checked, and furnished with the best fuel, will last much longer than will a machine that is neglected or maltreated. The same is true of the human organism. Proper nutrition, exercise, intellectual growth, the avoidance of harmful practices such as the use of tobacco products or drugs, or abuse of alcohol, appropriate health care, and living in a healthful environment are all factors that contribute to longevity or long life.

A full 80 percent of all deaths occur after age 65. People over the age of 85 are now the fastest growing segment of the population. Dementia, arthritis, diminished hearing and visual acuity, incontinence, and hip fracture all continue to occur at the same age as they did in the past. The chronic, non-fatal disorders of longevity destroy the quality of life and drain society's resources. Through appropriate prevention and intervention strategies, it is possible to defer disease and to minimize dysfunction.

There are basically two ways of increasing life expectancy. The first is through health promotion and disease prevention. The second is through broader and intensified research efforts, including the findings of molecular and cellular biology. It is probably more helpful to the older population to apply existing information, and to educate them to its beneficial effects. It is abundantly evident that exercise through aerobic activity and resistance training reduces physical frailty, but there is a reluctance on the part of older persons to engage in physical activity. Listed among the top ten causes of death are pneumonia and its complications, but the majority of persons over the age of 65 do not receive the pneumococcal vaccine. Although many older persons die of the flu in an epidemic, approximately half of the persons age 65 and over get a flu shot in the fall. Cancer of the lung has surpassed breast cancer in women, but smoking among women continues to increase, particularly among younger age groups. Diseases related to tobacco use and alcohol abuse continue to be the primary factors in premature death involving heart disease and cancer. In addition, older Americans continue to consume high fat diets, even though such foods have been clearly demonstrated to increase the incidence of heart disease and cancer.

The delay of dysfunction means reduction both in the length and the amount of dependency. The redundancy of various bodily systems and their capability to repair themselves are underlying factors for the biological basis of the mechanism of delay. Caloric restriction has shown to delay dysfunction and to even ward off death. Gene regulation is key to controlling a wide panorama of potential dysfunction. Stress reduction is increasingly associated with treatments for brain disorders, including Alzheimer's disease.

Aging research at all levels is essential to lower disability rates and to lengthen life. Additional years of life spent bedfast or in an institutional setting are not the anticipated rewards of long life. While it is accepted that aging contributes to increased vulnerability to disease and disability, it is vital to understand what precedes or leads to particular types of dysfunction. The three major precursors to disease which can be significantly altered through extensive research efforts include genetics, aging, and the environment. To postpone dysfunction may, in the case of aging, carry greater significance than the possibility for cure.

Age Categories

As the population continues to age, there is the realization that the elderly have been too globally perceived and that demarcations as to age groups are exceedingly important if this group is to be served appropriately. Unfortunately, a number of euphemisms continue to be employed in describing the older population, and researchers have used terms which, in some cases, have bordered on the esoteric.

Language directly affects behaviors. If persons are referred to in negative ways, there is a tendency to ignore such individuals and to provide less well for them. This, unfortunately, is also true of aging. The disparaging terms used to describe this age group include terms such as golden agers, senior citizens, old fogies, old geezers, and crocks. Such labeling, by and large negative, has hampered society's ability to deal effectively with the older population both conceptually and scientifically.

Researchers have confounded their studies by dividing older persons into amorphous categories such as the "young old," "the old old," "oldest old," "the frail elderly," "the well elderly," and the "long-living." Others have facetiously referred to older age groups as the "slow go," the "no-go," and the "go-go;" or simply "the risky" and "the frisky."

Unfortunately, such stereotyping of older persons persists in spite of the fact that dictionary terms have been available which adequately describe older age groups. Most people until they reach age 70 are not markedly different from other age groups. A proper terminology would include:

Septuagenarians	70 – 79
Octogenarians	80 – 89
Nonagenarians	90 – 99
Centenarians	100 – 109
Centedecinarians	110 – 119
Centeventenarians	120 – 129
Centetrentenarians	130 – 139

The last three appellations are neologisms coined to meet modern exigencies to properly define older age groups. A further advantage to the use of such nomenclature is that these terms have a Latin base and allow for international comprehension of their use to describe particular age groups.

It is clear that terms such as "the elderly" do not sufficiently distinguish between the age groups, particularly since there is a vast difference between the health, physical functioning, and health or social services required by septuagenarians and centenarians which spans a 30-year interval. Unfortunately, for too long, everyone over the age of 65 has been labelled elderly, and it is only now patently clear that such a distinction is practically meaningless.

Appropriate terminology is important in scientific investigations, in the clinical study of geriatrics, in assessing the needs of persons, and in ascribing clarity to specifically what group of persons is under discussion.

Research on Old Age

There is yet to develop a level of scientific information requisite to an appropriate study of aging and the processes of aging. There is currently a lack of information regarding many of the diseases which people suffer in old age. Lack of interest in the diseases of the elderly has long prevailed. Until fairly recently, autopsies were not routinely performed on older patients. The disinterest in the elderly extended to a disinterest in knowing of what they had died. Death certificates frequently listed as the cause of death "old age." Research on aging was not seriously undertaken until after World War II.

The increase in the aging of the population led to the realization that as people lived longer, they also used more health care services due to the increased incidence of disease and disability. From a purely economic standpoint, the importance of scientific research to uncover preventive measures spurred the establishment of centers for the study of aging.

The principal study that has been conducted in the United States is the Baltimore Longitudinal Study conducted by the National Institutes of Health on the male population. The study of women, despite the fact that women have historically lived longer than men, was instituted much later.

Much of the information available on aging has been derived from animal studies. Such information, however valuable, has its limitations. There is a danger in extrapolating information based on animal studies and to then apply this information to the human species. The shorter life expectancy of many animals makes them easier to study as they can be followed from birth to death, and, also, scientific experimentation on animals is permissible.

Demography

A proper assessment of population growth and change is vital to proper planning for the needs and concerns of society. Demography is the study of such population changes and their impact on the broader society. Such studies are particularly significant when such changes affect the nature of human experiencing because of age changes and population shifts and the provision of services to match such population changes.

One such change which has decided ramifications for health care services is that the sector of the population that is aged 85 and older is growing at a rapid rate. This population group also suffers from multiple health problems and occasions greater costs in terms of health expenditures. Research on maintaining health in old age is also of economic interest in order to offset costs of hospitalization and long-term care. The major emphasis in long-term care is now in skilled nursing facilities. Whereas long-term care had been characterized by various levels, its principal focus now is on the provision of skilled care. People admitted to skilled nursing facilities are in their eighties or older and generally require total care. The development of retirement centers, home health care, and the general overall improvement of health in older persons has led to such changes.

Technology: The Practical Application of Science

The practical application of science can be at either the levels of high technology or low technology. On occasion, simple solutions, on the level of low technology have more practical outcomes.

Some high technology streams, such as genetics, robotics, informatics, and communication technology provide the potential for very powerful and controversial applications. The science of genetics is leading to the possibility of predicting such conditions as heart disease and Alzheimer's disease.

In industrial applications, robotics has meant freeing labor from unwanted repetitive tasks, as well as freeing up labor for more important tasks. Such applications of robotics can be used to meet human needs, as well. The most important feature of the application of robotics so far is that it has provided a certain amount of dignity for the individual who is helped. It offers the promise of being able to do things for oneself that normally require a caregiver to perform. For example, fetch-and-carry systems could routinely deliver various supplies to the rooms of some nursing home residents. A robotic system, Helpmate, is being used in hospitals to deliver late trays and to perform errands.

Communication is probably the most important feature of human experience—removing isolation and preventing depression. Although most of today's elderly have had little experience with computers, the evidence, though scant, indicates that they are receptive to using the new technology, either "as is" or when tailored to their needs. The elderly of the future are likely to be more open to using computers because of exposure to them throughout their lifetimes.

Computer-Assisted Health Instruction

The use of computer-assisted health instruction is a logical extension of self-care and self-help. The growing use of information technologies for educating the public about maintaining health and preventing or treating disease is rapidly increasing the number of software programs on health education and management.

The relevance of this technological phenomenon for use by and for the elderly has not yet been widely recognized in either the private or public sector; however, the use of information technologies, particularly the microcomputer, could help the elderly maintain independent living, and is likely to be particularly effective when used in conjunction with physicians and other health care providers.

Future computer use by patients is expected to reach beyond providing them with information about their health status to become a virtual "hospital on the wrist." The concept of the hospital on the wrist includes a computer, a microminiature analyzer, and drug reservoirs with electronic probes capable of monitoring changes in the body, measuring vital signs, analyzing blood and enzymes, and comparing findings with expected values for the individual wearing it. The device would be able to communicate with computers of the wearer's physician as well as with computers in hospitals or other medical institutions and could administer drugs directly through the skin. It could also signal the patient when direct medical care was needed.

As envisioned, the hospital on the wrist does not offer the patient total medical autonomy but includes interactions between the patient, his or her computer, and the computers of health professionals. Computers and telecommunications now in use by patients for health purposes are oriented to assisting physicians and other health professionals with patient management in various health settings.

Computer-assisted health care that complements professional care may enable chronically ill people to remain in their homes when they wish to do so. A number of factors point to an increase in the proportion of the chronically ill population who may choose home care over institutional care in the future. Moreover, advances in medical technology now allow services to be provided at home that once required an institutional setting. Reductions in size and complexity have made many machines portable. Telecommunication equipment connecting patients and health professionals can facilitate their interaction and enhance the quality of care.

Other examples of medical technologies that can be connected to computers, thereby assisting health professionals with patient care, include analog signals from both mechanical and electrical devices that can be converted to digital signals for transmission to health professional computers.

"Smart" sensors–those incorporating microprocessors–currently sense and measure blood pressure, pulse rates, body temperature, and electrical activity of the heart. Measurements of other physical functions have been developed for use in rehabilitating handicapped patients; those that have the potential for computer-based processing may be applicable for monitoring the health status of segments of the older population.

Computer technology can enable hospital-based approaches for managing chronic diseases to be expanded to the home. A study of cirrhotic ambulatory patients found that they were able to systematically measure and communicate medically and behaviorally significant information.

Computers that monitor such household functions as turning on and off lights, radios, televisions, and providing wake-up service by voice synthesizers that speak preprogrammed messages, could be programmed to remind elderly persons of medication times, instruct them on diet and medical care practices, and remind them of physician and other health professional visits. Devices could be programmed to track medicinal intake and periodically dispense medicines. A bedside automated programmable dispensing machine has been developed for use in hospitals that may be adaptable for use in the home.

Society has rejected two of the most obvious remedies of the past, hiding the disability or hiding the disabled. Alternatives are now available in aids that are attractive, and that would be used without reservation, and, in some cases, even with pride.

Initially, technical aids were not always popular with the professionals in institutions and with society in general. Much work had to be done to create a degree of acceptance for the aids; it was easier in some cases than in others. The fact that many professional people are uncomfortable with technical devices and resist their introduction has been all too evident.

Technological advances in the medical-device area have had a profound impact on patient survival and improved quality of life. The benefits have been particularly notable for chronic diseases or dysfunctions that become more prevalent with increasing age.

The most significant contributions have been made in the area of implantable systems. These include intraocular lenses, heart valves, urethral sphincters, penile implants, cochlear implants, electrical pain control, cardiac pacemakers, defibrillators, artificial joints, and drug pumps. In each instance, the intent is to return the patient to a situation as close to normal as the state of the art permits. By virtue of their being implanted, these devices become relatively transparent to the patient. They tend to free the patient of the responsibility as well as the emotional involvement that may accompany their disease.

With the advent of visiting nurse associations, the older population can receive intravenous medications in a home setting instead of the hospital. This helps prevent environmental confusion in that companionship and security in familiar surroundings are available. Services such as homemakers allow older persons to maintain mobility in the household. Video and audio cassettes are helpful in rehabilitation. Large type is available in health instruction magazines and with medical instructions. National organizations such as the Arthritis Foundation, American Cancer Society, and others have grown significantly and help pave the way for the latest medical discoveries.

Medical Devices and Instrumentation for the Elderly

The human body is endowed from birth with many natural defenses, including autoimmunity and redundancy of tissues, organs, and parts, enabling it to resist the changes that come with age, disease, and trauma. As human beings age, such natural defenses gradually fail and may require replacements. The growing number of medical devices and instrumentation that has characterized modern health care may well substitute for loss of such natural defenses.

Today's medical devices can improve the functioning of, and in some instances replace, body parts that have deteriorated due to age or disease. Some examples include dental prostheses that are utilized in cases of tooth loss, hip prostheses and mechanical aids that help with problems of mobility.

Ethical dilemmas abound with respect to when, where, and how to implement such medical interventions. When would a person be considered too old to be given such a device? What is the rationale for keeping older persons alive when they suffer from irreversible brain disease or dementia? The responses to such questions become increasingly more complex as medical technology and science continue to advance and to provide alternative treatment possibilities. Technology now can control the timing and quality of individual demise.

Biological Aging

There are a number of older persons who function very well into advanced old age, and because of better life-style choices and increased income, educational level, and accessibility of new medical technologies, their number will continue to grow. Those who are well endowed with respect to genetic structure and have experienced the advantages of good health throughout the life span will very likely enjoy a healthy old age.

There are inevitable biological changes which occur as an individual becomes older. Such changes, however, are not the result of disease but are more aptly attributed to the aging process known as senescence. This term refers to the bodily changes that occur, and the limitations which such changes may impose. This term is not to be confused with the world "senile" which is often used as a pejorative term to describe older persons who may be suffering from physical or mental dysfunctions.

There are some diseases which are more likely to occur as a person continues to age. This does not mean that persons will necessarily suffer from such diseases. Diseases which may have had their onset in early periods of life manifest themselves as persons live to reach advanced old age. Such diseases can be the result of unhealthful lifestyles followed by the individual for a number of years. Cancers and diseases of the circulatory system are among those that manifest themselves in old age. The use of a number of medications to treat the multiple chronic diseases sometimes suffered by older persons can also lead to additional health problems. Drug dosages and uses have not been sufficiently studied in old age.

Biological Systems

Although the systems within the body are described as separate systems, they do not operate independently but often share or complement bodily functions. They are treated as separate systems in order to understand their functioning for didactic purposes. They are, however, intimately interconnected. For example, what happens to the respiratory system can affect the digestive system, which, in turn, can affect the general balance of the organism or the homeostasis of the body.

REFERENCES

Andrews, G.R. (Ed). (1998). Ageing beyond 2000: One world one future. *Australian Journal on Aging, 17*(1), Supplement.

Butler, R.N., & Brody, J.A. (Eds.). (1995). *Delaying the Onset of Late-Life Dysfunction.* New York: Springer.

Coombs, F. (1994). Engineering technology in rehabilitation of older adults. *Experimental Aging Research, 20,* 201-209.

Evers, M., Townsend, C., & Thompson, J. (1994). Organ Physiology of Aging. *Surgical Clinics of North America, 74* (1), 23-39.

Fries, J.F. (1980). Aging, natural death, and the compression of morbidity. *New England Journal of Medicine, 303,* 125-130.

Harris, R. (Ed.). (1983). *Medical devices and instrumentation for the elderly.* Arlington, VA: Association for the Advancement of Medical Instrumentation.

Haug, M.R. (1994). Elderly patients, caregivers, and physicians: Theory and research on health care triads. *Journal of Health and Social Behavior, 35,* 1-12.

Howell, S. (1994). The potential environment: Home, technology and future aging. *Experimental Aging Research, 20,* 285-290.

Klerk, M., Huijsman, R., & McDonnell, J. (1997). The use of technical aids by elderly persons in the Netherlands: An application of the Andersen and Newman Model. *The Gerontologist, 37* (3), 365-373.

Lesnoff-Caravaglia, G. (Ed.). (1987). *Aging in a Technological Society.* New York: Human Sciences Press.

Lesnoff-Caravaglia, G. (Ed.) (1988). *Handbook of Applied Gerontology.* New York: Human Sciences Press.

Oram, J.J. (1997). *Caring for the Fourth Age.* London: Armelle.

McConnel, E., & Murphy, E. (1990). Nurses' use of technology: An international concern. *International Nursing Review, 37,* (5), 331-334.

Quivery, M. (1990). Advanced medical technology: Finding the answers. *International Nursing Review, 37* (5), 329-331.

Ross, I. K. (1995). *Aging of Cells, Humans & Societies.* Dubuque, IA: Wm. C. Brown Publishers.

Rowe, J. W., & Kahn, R. (1996). *Successful Aging.* New York: Pantheon.

Stolley, J., & Buckwalter, K. (1991). Iatrogenesis in the elderly. *Journal of Gerontological Nursing, 17* (9), 30-34.

Chapter 2

THE INTEGUMENTARY SYSTEM
- outward signs of aging

The more obvious signs of aging are external and are physically observable, such as the graying of hair, the wrinkling of skin, or stooped posture. Such outward signs of aging do not necessarily indicate the level of energy or activity of which the individual may be capable. Because the integumentary system is a highly visible system, it frequently affects the social, psychological, and economic aspects of a person's life.

Heredity

Heredity plays a major role in when people age, the rate of aging, and which bodily systems will be most affected by senescence. Some persons begin to gray in their late teens, while others never experience graying of the hair. Predispositions toward certain diseases may begin to manifest themselves as the individual grows older, and disease states can cause alterations in the integumentary system. Changes can also result from particular medical interventions and treatments.

The Skin and General Health Status

The integumentary system is often taken for granted. People show little concern for the skin unless they become sunburned or experience itching or some other discomfort. The skin, however, is an important indicator of the general state of health of the individual. Some cancers are first noted when the skin presents with an unusual appearance; these cancers may actually have their locus in some other internal organ such as the pancreas, but its early indications appear on the surface of the skin. Geriatric physicians frequently make it a practice to examine the skin surface for such indications.

Due to extreme exposure of the skin during occupational or recreational activities, the skin can be affected by photoaging which can also result in skin cancers. In spite of our cavalier treatment of the skin, the skin plays an important function in protecting the body against onslaughts from the environment. The skin plays an important role in maintaining the homeostasis of the body. The integumentary system involves the entire surface of the body through skin, hair or nails.

The first reaction to the environment is reflected through the skin. The sensing of heat or cold causes the body to approach or to withdraw. Sweat glands important to the maintenance of appropriate body temperature are located in the skin. The skin also serves as a barrier to prevent the intrusion of foreign substances into the body such as toxins or poisons. It serves as a protection against the bites of insects and the infiltration of microorganisms. The skin, however, is a useful surface for the administration of certain medications because of their easy absorption through the skin.

With aging, there is a change in the texture and general appearance of the skin. The coloring of the skin also has an important role to play in offsetting the harmful effects of ultraviolet rays. People inhabiting different portions of the world exhibit a skin color adapted to their environment to ward off potential harmful environmental effects. In this regard, skin color serves as a protective device.

Along with the network of sweat glands, there is also a layer of blood vessels which help in the regulating of temperature and in the homeostasis of the body. When the body temperature rises, the blood vessels dilate, they spread out to provide more blood closer to the surface of the skin. The moisture provided by the sweat glands covers the surface of the body which is then evaporated, and the body is cooled. In older persons this temperature regulating system operates less efficiently, and this explains, in part, why when temperatures rise, there is an increase in the incidence of older persons suffering from heat stroke or dying.

The skin also provides significant information to the brain, so that the body knows how to act or to react. Heat, cold, or sensitivity to pain and touch are relayed to the brain through the skin. The skin is able to absorb various drugs and compounds, much as does the liver. Since the skin surface reacts easily to drug absorption, it is used to counteract illness such as motion sickness or to alter smoking habits. Skin patches are effective because the skin can absorb the chemical compounds that make up the drug. Anything that passes through the skin eventually enters the blood stream, and, consequently, does not need to be injected or taken orally. Furthermore, it provides a constant dosage for a long period of time. Thus, it is effective in a variety of treatment procedures. Use of the skin for treatment procedures is particularly important in dealing with older persons who may have difficulty in swallowing medications. The skin also plays a role in the immune system and helps in the growth and development of cells to offset the attacks of various foreign elements.

The uninterrupted covering provided by the skin provides protection to the body and is made up principally of two layers, the dermis and the epidermis. The skin layers over the body are not all uniform with certain portions having thicker layers than others. For example, the skin on the soles of the feet is thicker and on the palms of the hands. As a result of such layers of thickness, persons can develop calluses due to unusual thickening of the skin surface. The melanin or coloring of the skin is located in the epidermis, while the glands in the skin lie beneath in the dermis. Included are the oil or sebaceous glands which secrete the oils which lubricate the hands in particular and function to keep the body smooth to facilitate movement of fingers and limbs.

Because of its location on the body surface, the integumentary system is influenced by environmental factors as well as by changes within the body. Wrinkles and sagging skin appear, and the skin tends to become thinner, less pliable, and dryer. There is a generalized loss of fat from the hypodermis beneath the skin, which, coupled with diminished elasticity, causes the skin to become loose, and folds and wrinkles become prominent. Fat loss causes the body framework to become more obvious, which can give an emaciated appearance to some older persons.

Although the number of pigment-producing cells diminishes significantly with age, those remaining move closer together to form dark age spots. Nails become thicker and curved, while growing more slowly. There is a generalized loss of hair, and the remaining hair tends to lose its color and to appear gray.

The integumentary system comprises the skin, hair, nails, and various glands located in the skin. All of these components help maintain a stable internal environment (homeostasis) within the body so that the various cells composing the body are able to function normally.

Epidermis

The superficial portion of the skin is the epidermis. The epidermis is generally quite thin, but it can increase in thickness in areas where there may be unusual pressure or friction. Two such bodily surfaces are the soles of the feet and the palms of the hands. Prolonged pressure can result in the formation of calluses or corns. The color of the skin is determined primarily by the pigment called melanin located within the epidermis. Varying amounts of melanin determine skin color. Large amounts result in darker skin color, lesser amounts produce yellow or white skin.

Dermis

Directly beneath the epidermis lies the dermis which contains sweat glands and oil-secreting sebaceous glands. The secretions of the sebaceous glands provide the lubrication for the epidermis to allow for smoother movements, particularly in areas such as the fingers. The blood vessels of the dermis are responsible for the reddish tint of the skin of light skin races.

Information regarding environmental stimuli which lead to sensations of touch, pressure, pain, and temperature changes are provided to the nervous system through specialized receptors.

Aging and the Integumentary System

The changes that occur in the skin with age are not what might be described as life-threatening. Despite such changes, the health of the person is not seriously compromised. The skin gradually becomes thinner with age, and the number of immune cells in the skin diminishes. The skin can become more susceptible to chemical irritants.

Due to water and fat composition changes, the skin can begin to assume the characteristics of aging. The skin begins to wrinkle and sag. Scales or uneven patches of rough skin may appear, or growths on the skin itself. The skin surface is prone to crack or break easily.

Sweat glands and sebaceous glands are gradually reduced in number. As a result, older persons tend to sweat less, and their skin can become dry and parchment-like. An additional consequence of the reduction in sweat glands and the inability to perspire, is that older persons are less able to regulate body temperature. Such inefficient body temperature regulation can lead to heat exhaustion. Caution with regard to exposure to the sun also becomes significant due to such reductions in function. Older persons should also be encouraged to drink increased amounts of water. Because of the generalized reduction in blood flow to the skin, the skin surface of older persons may appear cooler than in younger individuals. Compromised thermoregulation makes the older person more susceptible to hyperthermia (heat exhaustion) and hypothermia (reduced body temperature). Hypothermia can be life-threatening.

The growth of the fingernails and toenails is compromised by the lowered skin temperature and may grow more slowly. Nails may become brittle, and crack or break easily. Due to deposition of calcium, the fingernails and toenails may become discolored and thicker, and to develop ridges. There may be curving of the toenails. Such changes are particularly problematic for women whose cosmetic care often includes painting and attention to the fingernails and toenails.

Due to the reduced sensitivity to pain, the older person may not be aware of having stepped on a sharp object, such as a tack or piece of glass. Infections can lead to problems of immobility, or to even more serious consequences for people who are diabetic.

Attention to foot problems is vital to older persons as lack of care can result in reduced mobility and dependence. The assistance of a podiatrist who specializes in care of the feet can be sought before problems become serious. Podiatrists can also recommend special shoes or shoe alterations to accommodate foot problems. Many institutions have arrangements by which podiatrists make regular visits to residents, and there are podiatrists, much like dentists, who have traveling units equipped to care for patients in various locations.

Evidence of the biological process of aging occurs throughout the body, including the feet. Toenails become thicker and generally discolored. The skin becomes dryer. Calluses, corns and bunions occur more commonly.

NAILS. Many older individuals are unable to easily reach their feet because of obesity, arthritis or dizziness. In addition, their eyesight is often poor. As the toenails become thicker, they are more difficult to trim.

Nails can often become ingrown, on one or both sides of the nail. This can result in pain, redness, swelling, and infection. Depending on the extent of involvement and the patient's vascular status, one border or the entire nail can be removed. If the problem is recurrent and the patient is a suitable candidate, part or all of the nail can be removed on a more permanent basis by chemical or surgical means.

BONE STRUCTURE CHANGES. Many older persons experience pain in the joints of their feet which is often caused by arthritis, along with normal wear and tear. These patients usually benefit from molded shoes. Surgery may also be considered, dependent on adequate vascular status.

CORNS AND CALLUSES. These are an accumulation of dead skin cells caused by underlying bony prominence and friction from shoegear. Treatment consists of regular visits to the podiatrist for debridement and padding. For some patients, the option of surgical correction can be considered.

HAMMERTOES. The "buckling" of smaller toes, caused by a muscle imbalance or shoes that are too short, is referred to as hammertoes. Pain occurs from corns on the top of the toes. Treatment consists of debridement, protective padding, extra-depth shoes, or surgery.

BUNIONS. A bunion is an excessive bony bump on the inside of the foot, near the great toe joint. This can cause problems in wearing shoegear. Bunions are usually a result of pronation ("flattening" of the feet) and may have a hereditary component. Treatment consists of wide shoes, orthotic devices, bunion shields, and surgery.

WARTS. Warts are caused by a virus. Plantar warts occur on the soles of the feet. Many different treatment modalities exist, from padding and using a weak acid solution, to surgical excochleation.

NEUROMAS. Impingement of a nerve between two metatarsal bones can lead to "shooting" pain to the toes and enlargement of the nerve, or neuroma. This pain is usually aggravated by tight shoegear. Treatment includes injections, orthotic devices with accommodations, and surgical excision.

POOR CIRCULATION. With advancing age, circulation to the extremities usually decreases. The effects of decreased circulation are often first seen in the feet, because they are the farthest part of the body from the heart. The skin may become dry and more susceptible to infection. Varicose veins and numbness may also be experienced. Support hose can be helpful for the circulation. Lotions or creams can be applied to moisturize the skin, particularly after bathing. Depending on the extent of the circulatory problem, patients are often referred to a vascular specialist for further evaluation.

Hair

There is a generalized loss of body hair, particularly on the head. Men and women with a genetic predisposition toward baldness will find an increase in hair loss with age. There is a reduction in the presence of body hair overall, including the underarm and pubic areas. On some parts of the body there appears to be an increase in the proliferation of hair. This is particularly true of older men. They experience extensive growth of hair in the nostrils and ears. The hair in the eyebrows, not only grows longer, but can also extend in different directions. Women may experience an increase in facial hair with the growth of a mustache or beard. Removal of such hair growth is easily accomplished through a variety of cosmetic procedures.

One of the most obvious age changes is a change in the color of the hair. There is a gradual reduction of pigment in the hair with aging, resulting in a loss of hair color. For some women, the graying of the pubic hair is viewed with alarm and is taken as a sign of growing older. Heredity may play a role in the amount of hair color lost and at what age the change occurs. Some people gray prematurely, as early as the mid-twenties, while others do not experience change in hair color until advanced old age. The hair coloring which is a mixture of dark and gray, resulting in the salt and pepper effect, is hair that still retains some pigment. The very white hair that is sometimes seen in persons in their seventies or eighties is hair from which pigment is totally absent.

There appears to be a reduced sensitivity to touch. In regions of the skin that are not covered by hair, there are also indications of a decline in the sensitivity of temperature receptors. As a result, persons can be burned by touching extremely hot objects, such as cooking utensils. The finer sensations of touch such as the smoothness or roughness of surfaces seems to diminish, as well as responses to textures such as silk or satin. There is some indication that older persons experience a decreased sensitivity to pain. Older persons have been treated in emergency rooms for the extraction of pins and needles from the feet which, until infected, had caused minor discomfort.

Hypodermal Changes

The hypodermis located just beneath the skin exhibits a generalized loss of fat from the subcutaneous tissue. This loss is usually most obvious in the face and the limbs. The loss of subcutaneous fat is a major cause of wrinkles and is responsible for the emaciated appearance of some older persons. It also results in a loss of body padding which allows bony prominences to protrude causing discomfort and potential skin problems.

The gradual loss of subcutaneous fat also means that the body is less well insulated, and that greater amounts of body heat escape. Due to the loss of fat and diminished blood supply to the skin, older persons may require warmer environments to feel comfortable.

The protective aspects of the integumentary system are compromised as persons age. The thinning or lack of hair interferes with its heating and cooling function, while the reduction in fat eliminates the body's protective padding. The loss of sweat glands affects thermal regulation, and the loss of oil glands diminishes facile movement.

Dysfunctions

Decubitus Ulcers

Decubitus ulcers, or pressure sores, usually occur in people who are bedfast for long periods of time or are immobilized. People who utilize wheelchairs for extended periods of time are also subject to this condition. In older persons, this is a common problem due to the generalized loss of fat that consequently exposes bony structures. Furthermore, since the circulatory system is less efficient in old age, there is a reduction in blood supply to the skin. These are the primary factors that predispose older persons to develop pressure sores.

The sores generally develop in areas where the skin is under constant pressure, such as hips or heels. Leaning on one side for long periods of time or resting on an elbow can result in the development of pressure sores. Remaining in one position for a long period time and the rubbing of the skin against sheets and blankets all serve to irritate the skin. Pressure sores can result in lesions so deep that craters develop in the skin exposing bone and tissue. With proper care and treatment, the sores can be eliminated, but the problem can reoccur due to the immobility of the patient. There is further the danger of infection. Improving nutritional levels can also be beneficial in treatment programs.

Turning of the patient and constant surveillance are important. Care of patients whose treatments require prolonged bed rest, such as those on respirators or residents in long-term care facilities, can become particularly problematic. This is a concern with respect to the rapidly growing age 85 and older group who are more often hospitalized and utilize long-term care facilities.

The use of special bed mattresses made of materials which allow for a more responsive give to the weight of the person can also serve to ameliorate the problem. Such mattresses have been developed using water, spun glass, air, or plastic materials. Preventive health measures that ensure against prolonged immobility probably are the best forms of intervention.

Lentigo

Lentigo is a condition in which darkened areas appear on flat areas of the aging skin. These dark brown spots are usually seen on the backs of the hands and on the face. They are caused by an increased deposition of melanin. They may also be found on the neck and chest. Although they have no tendency to become malignant, these dark spots gradually increase in size and become even darker with advancing age.

Skin changes include not only changes of pigmentation, but growth of skin layers which resemble scales and the development of skin tags that protrude from the skin itself and are usually found on the neck, under the breasts or armpits or generalized over the chest area. Wart-like growths and raised areas resembling birthmarks can also appear on the face, frequently in the area of the nose. Such changes also can be removed surgically or through topical applications and usually are benign. The appearance of such skin alterations can be variously attributed to the malfunctioning of the immune and endocrine systems in old age.

Senile Pruritus

With the loss of oil-secreting and sweat glands, there is a reduction in the water content of the skin as well as its motility. This causes the skin to become drier and less resilient. This results in breaks or tiny cracks in the skin or senile pruritus (itching). Because the skin itches, it causes people to scratch the area, bringing about further skin damage. Environmental factors can also add to the problem, such as high temperatures or strong wind. Frequent bathing also serves to dry the skin and can worsen the condition.

Skin color seems to play a role in the number of skin diseases to which the person may become subject. Light-skinned fair-haired persons appear to suffer more from such disorders than do persons who have darker skin and are dark-haired.

Herpes Zoster *¿ Tuberculosis (die dormant in the body)*

Herpes zoster is more frequently associated with younger persons. When it occurs in older persons, it is frequently referred to as "shingles." A disease common to persons between the ages of 50 to 70, its incidence generally tapers off and is rarely seen in individuals over the age of 70.

The virus responsible for shingles is also thought to cause chicken pox. As chicken pox, the virus enters the body and then remains dormant for many years. As the person ages, the virus becomes activated.

The person first experiences uncomfortable sensations such as itching and pain following the path of the affected nerves, down the spine and toward the chest. Small blister-like formations appear along these nerve pathways. Once the blisters dry, dark brown spots form over these areas. The disease and its attendant pain may last for several weeks or months.

Skin Cancer

While cancers of the skin are fairly common, early detection can result in successful treatment. Skin cancers need not be life-threatening. Due to the nature of their occupations, many men who work out-doors develop skin cancers. Since men have historically been reluctant to utilize health care services, procrastinating the receiving of medical attention when ill, this often leads to complications which early intervention might have alleviated. The shorter life expectancy of men is partly attributable to their reluctance to admit to illness and to avoid health care intervention. Women, on the other hand, possibly because of childbearing and greater responsibilities for their children's health, utilize health care services more readily, and, thus, are more likely to seek medical attention at earlier stages of illness such as cancer. Women, also, are less likely to be in occupations that place them in contact with the outside elements and, thus, avoid extensive exposure.

Life-threatening or malignant cancers can originate in the epidermis or the dermis, or can be associated with glands of the skin. Cancers that are not malignant and are not life-threatening are benign. Although any change in the appearance of a wart or a mole should be carefully followed, most cancers of the skin are not malignant.

The most common form of skin cancer is associated with exposure to sunlight. It occurs most frequently in light-skinned races because of their susceptibility to the damaging effects of excessive exposure to sunlight. Certain older vocational groups are particularly vulnerable, such as farmers and construction workers.

Secondary Skin Cancer

Some cancers which are detected in the skin can actually have their origin in other parts of the body. As these cancers spread to the skin, they are referred to as secondary cancers. Such cancers often appear on the skin directly over the site where the primary cancer is located.

The evidence of secondary skin cancers are generally found in middle-aged persons over the age of 50. They are frequently ignored, and little attention is given them simply because they usually do not present with symptoms. Their importance, however, is significant as the diagnosis of a secondary skin cancer may lead to the uncovering of a previously undiscovered primary cancer.

Aging changes in the integumentary system occur at different rates in different individuals. Factors that have an influence on the rate of aging include heredity, dietary habits, environmental factors, occupation and recreational preferences.

Prevention and Intervention through Technology

Plastic or Cosmetic Surgery

The societal attitude that places a high premium on looking and acting young means that the process of aging, as well as aged persons, are often viewed in a negative light.

Plastic or cosmetic surgery is a method commonly resorted to in order to obviate the signs of aging and to restore an image of youth. Plastic surgery can be performed on virtually all parts of the body, as well as the face. Both men and women resort to such treatment. Removal of wrinkles, altering facial structure, removal of unwanted pouches or sagging skin are some of the alterations sought. Breasts, hips, thighs, arms and legs can all be altered through surgery. For both sexes, the removal of fat through liposuction is a common procedure, as is hair replacement caused by baldness. Some areas of the body are more easily altered than others, and some procedures when repeated too frequently can create problems in health or appearance. The cost of such interventions has diminished, and, as a result, cosmetic surgery is more and more available to even the less affluent groups within the population.

The emphasis in American society upon looking young and attractive has spurred the use of cosmetic surgery for economic security. This is particularly true in some fields such as sales or entertainment. The negative stereotyping of older persons, particularly females, is probably the major reason why women resort to such interventions. The signs of aging may have negative psychological effects upon some persons, and surgical intervention may be viewed as having a therapeutic value.

As the population continues to age, marriages between generations are becoming commonplace. Both older men and women marry or develop relationships with much younger partners. As a result, when there is disparity in age between couples, and, consequently, one partner ages more rapidly than the other, cosmetic surgery is often the sought remedy.

When female attractiveness is based on meeting the correct fashion criterion for beauty, woman of all ages strive to achieve such an ideal. Through the influence of television commercials, people long to belong to the Pepsi® generation and to vacation in Marlboro® country.

Plastic surgery can provide a more youthful appearance, but it does not delay the aging process. Various creams and hair dyes help to disguise some aging changes.

Mobility and Independence Aids

The importance of proper footcare on aging and mobility cannot be overemphasized. Pedal problems, if left untreated, can lead to a decrease in walking or general activity. This, in turn, can create an increase in cardiovascular problems, and to a decrease in circulation and muscle tone.

Diabetics with proper instructions, footcare, and positive attitudes can often improve lower extremity maintenance and thus possibly avoid amputation. Arthritic deformities can be modified with minor surgical procedures and resilient footwear.

Often orthotic devices and jogging and walking shoes can arrest certain deformities. Some accommodative devices help to distribute weight from painful areas to healthier regions of the foot. Visually impaired persons often suffer from dermavision. The distal digits act as "antennae" in an attempt to combat the loss of vision. Such advances in mobility are extremely important because without mobility or foot health nearly every body system deteriorates.

Advances have been made in the use of mobility aids, such as crutches, canes, portable walkers, as well as answering devices, such as the wireless telephones.

Materials for shoegear and prosthetic/orthotic devices have improved primarily in the areas of flexibility and resilience, and have become increasingly lightweight. Tread sole of shoegear can increase walking safety in the winter months. Materials designed with perforation tend to decrease perspiration problems. Aerosols containing emollients, dermatological medications and powders obviate the need for bending over, and, hence, are of great value in geriatrics. Velcro on prosthetics and shoegear has been revolutionary for arthritics who are unable to tie laces easily. Artificial limbs have advanced beyond a functional basis. Care is taken to match the limbs so that shoe sizes will be the same for each limb.

Advances in technology regarding podiatric gerontology and foot health may be considered in three dimensions. The first is the detection and identification of these conditions with a degree of accuracy and timeliness; the second, with the added challenge in today's world of cost-effectiveness, treatment that is both economical and widely available; and, third, for patients under custodial care or in long-term care institutions, mobility and independence aids allow for the activities of daily living with minimal restriction and reduction of costs. The maintenance of mobility and activity adds both to the quality and length of life.

REFERENCES

Lesnoff-Caravaglia, G. (1988). *Aging in a Technological Society.* New York: Human Sciences Press.

Oram, J.J. (1997). *Caring for the Fourth Age.* London: Armelle.

Ross, I.K. (1995). *Aging of Cells, Humans & Societies.* Dubuque, IA: Wm. C. Brown Publishers.

Rowe, J.W., & Kahn, R. (1998). *Successful Aging.* New York: Pantheon.

Spence, A.P. (1995). *Biology of Human Aging* (2nd. ed.). Englewood Cliffs, NJ: Prentice-Hall.

Sunderkotter, C., Kalden, H., & Luger, T. (1997). Aging and the skin immune system. *ARCH Dermatology, 133,* 1256-1261.

Weinstock, M. (1997). Death from skin cancer among the elderly. *ARCH Dermatology, 133,* 1207-1209.

Chapter 3

THE SKELETAL AND MUSCULAR SYSTEMS

The Skeletal System

The skeletal system provides the structure for the body and can be thought of as a form of clothes hanger as everything is either draped or suspended over this framework. The skeleton is what gives the body its form.

The types of tissue that make up the skeletal system are bone and cartilage. Bones not only serve as structural support for the soft tissues of the body, but most of the body muscles are attached to bones. The skeletal system, through special movable joints, allows the body to move in a variety of ways.

The skeletal system also provides a protective function. Many of the internal vital organs of the body are housed in or are surrounded by bony structures. The brain and the spinal cord are protected by the skull and the vertebral column. The rib cage effectively surrounds the heart and the lungs. Such protective functions can be easily provided by bone because it is very hard and resilient.

Minerals that are significant for many body functions are also found in the bone. Such minerals include calcium, sodium, phosphorous and potassium. Another important function of the skeletal system is the formation of blood cells.

Changes in the skeletal system with age can have profound implications with respect to a persons's life-style. Mobility may be compromised due to the stiffening of joints and pain associated with the initiation or carrying out of even simple movements. Standing erect or maintaining an upright posture may be difficult due to structural changes in the vertebral column. Since bones become more brittle and fragile with age, the protective functions of the skeletal system may be diminished. People do not necessarily have to experience a fall to break a bone; brittle bones crush easily in a movement as simple as turning the body from one side to another. The breaking of a hip, for example, can have serious consequences for an older person. Such an individual may move from an independent life-style to placement in a nursing home setting. The breaking of a hip bone may have rendered it impossible for the person to continue to function adequately within the home environment. Such changes are psychologically damaging as well as physically debilitating, since most older persons prefer living in their own homes for as long as possible.

Such changes, however, vary in degree among individuals. Such age-related alterations in the skeletal system can be offset by appropriate exercise programs and the establishment of balanced nutritional practices over the life-span.

Bone

Bones vary in shape according to the exigencies of the body and are short, flat, irregular, and long. New bone continues to be formed as old bone is broken down, or resorbed, throughout life. The continuous cycle of formation and resorption of bone replaces the old and more brittle matrix, and remodels the bones to match the bodily needs over time. For example, when people gain weight their bones will become thicker and stronger to meet the changed bodily requirements.

Bone is also capable of undergoing structural changes that cause it to become stronger when subjected to stress. Older persons who lead sedentary lives, exercise less, or who spend long periods of time in bed due to illness, do not have this advantage. Movement is required for bone formation.

A major factor in the development of bone is proper nutrition. The consumption of vegetables is important to proper bone formation. Women begin to lose calcium from their bones as early as age 30. This is the age when many women begin to go on diets and to limit the amount of calcium they absorb. Such dietary changes hold more serious consequences for women than for men because women are more prone to diseases of the bone, such as osteoporosis. This disease results in porosity of the bones, and, although men are susceptible to this disease as well, it affects women at a higher rate, especially following menopause.

Older persons frequently do not follow a balanced diet. This may be due to loss of appetite, depression, or simply the condition of their teeth which makes chewing difficult. Many of the vegetables which harbor ingredients important to bone formation are eschewed by older persons because they have difficulty in masticating due to ill-fitting dentures or the total absence of teeth (edentulous). Dairy foods may be avoided because of lactose intolerance.

Cartilage

While the skeletal system is largely made up of bone, cartilage is important in terms of structural support and in the efficient movement of joints. Lack of exercise more often is the causative factor in the development of stiffness in joints. Sedentary life-styles are largely responsible for such stiffness.

Activities to prevent joint stiffness need not be strenuous. Gardening is an activity which is relaxing and causes persons to move about, to reach, and to stretch. Nursing homes, particularly in Europe, frequently provide gardens for residents that can be cared for from a variety of levels, from a reclining position, standing, or sitting in a wheelchair. People do not have to be excluded from activities because of a health problem or disability; the challenge lies in discovering new outlets that can continue to enhance life or ways to adapt the environment so as to meet the individual's new needs. Bedfast patients can also participate in exercises through activities geared toward their particular capabilities.

Dysfunctions

As persons age, the loss of calcium from bone is the major change in the skeletal system. Women experience such losses in greater severity than do men, with the amount of calcium in the bones steadily decreasing beginning at approximately the age of 30. For men, such losses in calcium are not initiated until the age of 60 or older. The rate of calcium loss can be reduced through regular participation in exercise programs.

The smooth functioning of the various movable joints of the body relies on the cartilage in the skeletal system. Joints are covered with an articular cartilage, which during movement, rub together. As people age, the cartilages of joints may become thinner, with the result that bone can rub against bone. Such changes can lead to pain and discomfort and can restrict the movement of the joint. Even movements like rising from a chair can be executed by some older persons with great difficulty. Unfortunately, once older persons encounter some difficulty in movement or experience some pain associated with such movement, they tend not to use that limb or that part of the body. Actually, they should be encouraged to continue the limb's use, but there is usually great resistance. It is disuse of the body that often creates problems of movement in old age. The body, by and large, is underused by most people.

As people grow older, there is a rigidity that takes place in the bone structure that can hamper movement. Some bodily functions can be affected by such alteration in bone structure. The respiratory system can function less efficiently because of the growing rigidity of the rib cage and reduced expansion of the lungs upon breathing. The inspiration and expiration of the lungs can be restricted.

There is a change in the intervertebral discs, and they begin to flattens causing persons to lose height. Persons are shorter in old age than when they were younger.

Bursitis

Inflammation of the joints becomes more common, especially among men, and often results in bursitis. Diagnoses of bursitis, however, should be carefully evaluated as the symptoms are similar to those for early signs of Parkinson's disease. Early detection of Parkinson's disease is crucial to the initiation of treatment procedures which are helpful only in the early stages. Such early detection is further complicated by the fact that men do not readily seek medical advice.

Arthritis

Arthritis is a major source of discomfort and disability for many older persons. It is one of the oldest known diseases. Arthritis is a general term that refers to various types of inflammation or degenerative changes that occur in joints. Arthritis is not limited just to older persons, but can afflict all age groups, including children.

The most important risk factor for arthritis is age. Other factors include: body type (risk is increased in stocky individuals, decreased in tall, thin people); risk is increased in Caucasians over African-Americans, Asians and Native Americans; diabetes (which may be partially controllable when due to obesity; and, genetic traits (one possible form is influenced by sex chromosomes; another involves many genes). Controllable risk factors include obesity and exercise. Many orthopedic surgeons fear that the current popularity of jogging and other vigorous exercises may exacerbate osteoarthritis. Overexercise can worsen the condition of those who have the disease.

The three most common types of arthritis are osteoarthritis (the most common), rheumatoid arthritis (second most common), and gouty arthritis.

Osteoarthritis

Osteoarthritis, also known as degenerative joint disease, is the most common joint disease. The second most common cause of disability, it affects some 50 million Americans. It is one of the most important causes of chronic disability, not only in the United States, but in other developed countries as well. The incidence of osteoarthritis rises with age, and because its prevalence increases as individuals live longer, it has become much more common in recent years. Some evidence of the disease has been found in 90 percent of people by age 40 (in autopsy studies). Symptoms become increasingly prevalent and more intense with age. This disease is so common that for many years it was considered a normal aspect of aging.

Osteoarthritis is the symptomatic disruption of joint function. It is marked by ulceration and destruction of joint cartilage, leading eventually to exposure and destruction of underlying bone. The normal cushioning effect of cartilage is lost, causing bone to rub on bone. Joints are fluid-filled spaces lined by cartilage and separating bones; those found on the limbs (legs and arms) are adapted to permit easy movement. Limb joints are most affected by this disease, especially those responsible for weight-bearing (hips and knees), the vertebrae, and (for unknown reasons) the joints closest to the tips of the fingers. The diagnosis of osteoarthritis is made by correlating symptoms of pain and stiffness with x-ray evidence of changes in joints. Inflamed joints are marked by pain, swelling, and decreased range of motion.

Arms and leg joints are composed of a fluid-filled cavity, surrounded by a fibrous capsule. The surfaces that move against one another are composed of cartilage. The cartilage sits over bone. The cartilaginous surfaces are extremely well adapted to ease of movement; they are four times as slippery as Teflon, one of the most frictionless artificial surfaces. Disruption of the health of the cartilage tissue can reduce this ease of movement, leading to joint stiffness. Irritation of surrounding tissues leads to the symptom of pain. Osteoarthritis is one of the causes of ill health of the joint cartilage.

Osteoarthritis is a chronic inflammation that causes the articular cartilages covering the ends of the bones in the affected joint to degenerate gradually. People often complain that their wrists hurt. Activities which were once enjoyable have to be foregone due to the excessive pain caused by joint movements. Knitting, playing tennis, or playing the piano are some of the forms of activities that people must forego. The loss of cartilage is not replaced, and this results in pain when joint movements are attempted. Joints continue to grow stiff over time, and in instances where the cartilage is missing, bone rubs against bone, causing intense pain. There are surgical interventions available to offset the loss of cartilage and to restructure the joint.

Excessive body weight, poor posture or repetitive job-related stresses (some forms of factory work or work on computers) are thought to contribute to the development of osteoarthritis. Heredity may be a factor. Its cause, however, is yet to be determined.

The Arthritis Foundation notes that patients with osteoarthritis wait an average of 4 years before seeking medical attention from a physician. This is unfortunate, because the progression of the disease can be retarded, and its symptoms ameliorated by routine treatments.

Although there is no cure for osteoarthritis, some simple interventions can greatly retard the progression of the disease. Use of a cane can, for example, reduce the stress placed on the hip during walking. Changing the environment by adapting beds and chairs for easier entry and exit, and arranging living space to avoid use of stairs can greatly diminish the demands on the individual and can minimize the need for movements that exacerbate the disease. Utensils and furniture that compensate for diminished function, especially of the hand and major joints of the legs, could greatly improve independent functioning. The design of computer keyboards need to be refined to make them accessible to those whose hand mobility is restricted by this disease.

The most common drug therapy is the use of high doses of aspirin. Extensive use of aspirin, however, can lead to hearing loss. Total joint replacement is a relatively new surgical technique made possible by technological advances in low-friction materials, biocompatible plastics and metals, and the development of cements that can function in bone. The joint most commonly replaced is the hip, but some centers are also performing knee replacement surgery, and surgery on other joints, such as fingers and shoulders, on an experimental basis. More than 60 percent of the total hip replacements done in the United States annually are done in those over 65. Hip replacement is now a routine procedure, which can reduce pain, improve mobility, and has a low risk of failure. All surgical procedures, however, must be carefully evaluated from individual perspectives, and, in some instances, may not be recommended.

New cases of rheumatoid arthritis decline after age 65. This condition is more common in women than in men and affects the small joints of the body such as those in the hands, feet, ankles, elbows and wrist. Chronic swelling of the joint causes the tendons that pass over the joint to be pushed out of their normal positions, thus causing deformity of the joint. People have difficulty in performing simple activities, and may have problems in feeding themselves. There appears to be a genetic link, although the exact cause is not fully understood. People who suffer this disease gradually experience marked declines in functional capacity.

Aspirin is frequently prescribed. Surgical intervention is often used in treating the affected areas or in replacing the diseased bone with a prosthetic device.

Gouty arthritis is considered an inherited condition caused by high levels of uric acid in the blood. It is found more frequently in men and in women following menopause. The areas usually affected include the big toe, the wrists, the elbows, the ankles, and the knees.

In older persons, however, certain medications may also increase uric acid levels. The inflammatory reaction is often first perceived in the big toe, but frequently includes other body joints. The common complaint is of morning stiffness and aching joints. Some persons have difficulty in getting out of bed in the morning and must have lift bars installed to assist them upon arising. For older persons this disease often creates dependency upon caregivers. This affliction has also long been linked to rich, fatty diets and an overuse of alcohol. Illustrations in old novels often picture an obese male character in a lounge chair with his stockinged foot perched on a foot stool with a wide bandage tied about the large toe.

Gouty arthritis is linked to life-style, as well as hereditary factors. People who suffer from gout can experience severe pain, not unlike walking on glass. Not only medications, but alterations in diet often seem to be of benefit.

Osteoporosis

Osteoporosis ("porous bone") is a major chronic disorder of older people, principally women following menopause. White and Asian women are at higher risk than Black women who tend to have greater bone density. A family history of osteoporosis also increases the risk of the disorder, as does a slight frame. Although men are subject to this disease, the disease, when contracted by men, seems to progress much more slowly than it does in women.

Osteoporosis is defined as a condition in which total bone mass is decreased while bone volume is unchanged; therefore, the density of the bone decreases. This thinning of the bone increases its fragility and makes it more susceptible to fracture. Activities and stresses that would not harm normal bone can result in fractures of osteoporotic bone. Loss of bone mass occurs in all people as they age, but the rate of loss is higher in women for about 10 years immediately following menopause. This period of rapid loss causes women to be especially subject to vertebral and wrist fractures.

This predisposition to fracture makes osteoporosis of significant importance to individuals over 40 and to the health care system. Diet is one of the major modifiable lifestyle factors which may affect progression of bone loss. The role of physical activity in preventing bone loss has yet to be determined.

Osteoporosis is an important cause of morbidity and mortality in the elderly. It appears to be the underlying cause of about two-thirds of hip fractures in older people. Osteoporosis is one of the commonest causes of back pain in older persons. The pain is due to the partial or complete collapse of a vertebra. Characteristically, the pain is very severe. Persons sometimes associate the onset of pain with pushing or lifting heavy weights, but it often starts spontaneously and has no definite precipitating, aggravating or relieving factors. The pain is difficult to control and potent analgesia is sometimes required.

Greater life expectancy and rising health care costs are expected to sharply increase the costs related to hip fractures. Fractures of the wrist are common, as are vertebral fractures. It is estimated that 25 percent of white women have at least one vertebral fracture by the age of 60. Most of these fractures are compression fractures or "crush fractures" in which the vertebra simply collapses from the weight of maintaining the body in the upright position.

Bone consists of a soft protein framework that is hardened by deposition of calcium salts. It is a dynamic tissue that is constantly being remodeled (reshaped and renewed) throughout a person's life. Bones provide the skeletal structure for the body and also serve as a repository of minerals such as calcium, magnesium, phosphorus, and sodium which are required for a variety of the body's functions. This remodeling of bone is accomplished by simultaneous resorption (removal of structural components) and formation (redeposition). Any condition in which resorption exceeds formation results in decreased bone mass. When women enter menopause, the rate of bone loss increases.

Treatment of osteoporosis is complex primarily because it involves care of problems arising from the underlying bone loss, that is fractures, and their sequelae. Hip fractures are a major occurrence; surgical repair of the fracture or replacement of the thigh is required. Surgical techniques and prosthetic devices have improved, and death rates now appear to be correlated more with age and predisposing disease than with common complications of surgery such as infections and embolisms. Total hip replacement is sometimes required. Fractures and the necessary immobilization following surgery further complicate the osteoporosis because lack of exercise results in further bone resorption and predisposes the individual to formation of clots in blood vessels. Carefully monitored estrogen therapy, calcium supplementation, vitamin D administration or exposure to sunlight, and exercise are all potentially effective methods of treatment. Vitamin D increases both bone resorption and formation. Hormone treatments may also prove effective in treating osteoporosis. However, calcium intake and absorption are widely accepted as important in preventing osteoporosis. Another critical element in maintaining bone health is exercise, specifically weight-bearing exercise.

Such loss of bone can result in diminished height, stooped posture, pain, and tooth loss. It can cause curvature of the spine and backache as vertebrae are eroded and compressed. The disease often causes a general reduction in the strength of bones, making them more easily fractured. Fracture and compression of the vertebrae produces the hunched back (widow's or dowager's hump) and shortening of the trunk. Because of the curvature of the spine, respiration can be adversely affected. Hip fractures are more common among older women.

There is as yet no consensus of opinion regarding the treatment of osteoporosis. A long-term diet deficient in calcium is considered to be a major contributing factor. Older persons are not able to absorb milk and other dairy products as well as younger persons. Hormonal changes associated with menopause—especially lowered estrogen secretion—are thought to be another major factor in its development. It is also more prevalent in people who are immobilized for prolonged periods of time. Residents of nursing homes are potentially susceptible. General difficulty in movement should be followed by a thorough physical examination to exclude the possibility of cancer that is finding expression through the skeletal system in impeding movement.

Estrogen therapy is an effective treatment for some women, but the dangers of such therapy which can lead to forms of cancer, lessens its broad scale use. Also, such therapy may not be indicated for all women following menopause.

Osteoporosis affects a significant number of elderly individuals. The morbidity and mortality associated with fractures are costly in terms of hospital care, long-term care, and rehabilitation, and the social costs to the individual and his or her family are substantial, although they cannot be precisely measured. Although research on bone physiology suggests the availability of preventive measures and treatments to those who are susceptible to osteoporosis, most preventive methods still require confirmation by research. Earlier diagnosis is considered important to a better prognosis, and such new technologies as photon absorptiometry make earlier diagnosis possible.

Osteoporosis is unlikely to be a single entity and probably includes several different pathogenic processes, all having a common endpoint: a reduced bone mass. There can be no single ideal treatment for all cases of osteoporosis.

Life-styles can be markedly changed by alterations in bone structure. Movement is decreased and general mobility is affected. Such gradual bodily disuse fosters the development of additional chronic disease, and, may, ultimately lead to death. Some skeletal changes are due to senescence. Others, however, are the result of life-style, including smoking.

Future Possible Interventions

There is increased attention being given to the potentially large market presented by an aging population for prosthetic devices. Companies that produce prosthetic devices could also greatly improve the functioning of arthritic individuals. Designers of chairs, stairways, beds, telephones, and computer keyboards are likely to continue to adapt their designs for use by the growing numbers of those affected by arthritis. Development of "smart" technologies to assist in daily activities should prove highly marketable to the large subpopulation.

A major problem in arthritis treatment is the proliferation of quack remedies and consumer fraud. The persistent and unremitting symptoms of pain and stiffness also make persons eager to seek remedies or any treatments that promise relief from such symptoms.

Prosthetic Joints for the Elderly

Limited motion and impaired activity are the bane of the elderly population. If impairment results from disease, and, if disability is the functional consequence of impairment, then handicap is the social consequence of disability. Stairs, revolving doors, heavy doors, high curbs, small curbs, low chairs, narrow passageways, tiny toilet booths, and all the other hazards impeding access and transportation conspire against those who have difficulty in moving. Together, these hazards and decrements disproportionately affect those with musculoskeletal or motor impairment, often to such a degree that they cannot experience the quality of life that is their due.

In an aged population, motion impairment usually results from one of two causes—stroke or arthritis. Because arthritis in its various forms is rarely fatal, patients suffering from arthritis grow old with the disease. The disease increasingly forces these individuals to limit their activities and opportunities in light of the architectural barriers and social problems specific to their group, thus causing an entire population group to be handicapped.

Osteoarthritis occurs chiefly in older persons as the consequence of prior injury or inflammation. Use, abuse, overuse or disease of a joint can, over time, sufficiently damage the joint to result in osteoarthritis. This lesion is a state of balance between destruction and repair. The loss of cartilage and the subchondral bone fractures represent the destructive aspects. The end result is limited motion. When this limited motion is accompanied by pain–and especially if this pain is also felt when the joint is immobile–the lesion often defies medical treatment. Various analgesic anti-inflammatory compounds can reduce the pain resulting from secondary inflammation, a common side effect of the disease, but can do little to alter the progress of the osteoarthritic lesion. Hips and knees are especially vulnerable to osteoarthritic changes.

Joint replacements have radically changed the outcome of locomotor dysfunction in the elderly. Most patients are able to walk without canes or crutches several months following the operation. Most patients report that pain is almost totally relieved and that the joint is functional, with its motion materially enhanced. An elderly person does not hold joints in the same position as a younger person. For example, many of the elderly have natural mild flexion stances of hips and knees. However, with appropriate postsurgery therapy, even these normal deficits can be overcome and gait can be returned to a premorbid state–in fact, to a state more closely resembling that of much younger persons.

Prosthetic replacement of various joints is a burgeoning industry. By reducing the amount of time needed for bed rest, by sparing the patient prolonged hospitalization that can lead to disorientation, by increasing the life span, and by decreasing the discomfort, these operations have been more successful than any other treatment in improving the quality of life for the elderly person who has locomotor impairment.

The Muscular System

As in the case of the skeletal system where there are numerous bones, varying in size to suit particular bodily functions, so there exist a variety of muscles to help execute bodily movements. Since the muscular system operates without any conscious decision on the part of the person, much like the integumentary system, the muscular system is taken for granted. People smile, walk, move about, blink their eyes, using a number of muscles without much regard to the complex coordination that permits such activity to occur. Muscles are constantly in use.

Changes in the muscular system can affect many parts of the body simultaneously, and can cause great inroads into a person's self-esteem. Body image is a very important factor in how individuals view themselves, and is an integral part of personal identity. The inability to perform certain movements as persons age can lead to serious depressive states.

The skeletal system and the muscular system are interminably linked. It is their dual coordinative functions that permit persons to move about easily and to perform small to gross movements.

There are over 600 muscles in the body of various sizes. The three types of muscle in the body are skeletal, smooth and cardiac. The structure of each muscle type is particular to its usage, and each muscle type is geared toward carrying out specific and unique functions.

The striped or striated skeletal muscle attaches to bones and causes all of the movements of the various joints. They can be voluntary—under the control of the individual—or involuntary—under the control of impulses conveyed to the muscle from the nervous system.

The muscle that is located in the walls of hollow organs and tubes such as the stomach, intestines, and blood vessels is smooth muscle. Through its contractions, smooth muscle regulates the passage of substances through various bodily structures. Smooth muscle is involuntary muscle and plays an important role in the digestive system.

The muscle associated with the heart is the cardiac muscle that forms the wall of the heart. It is striated or striped like skeletal muscle. The cardiac muscle, however, contracts involuntarily as does smooth muscle.

With aging, there is a gradual reduction in strength and endurance, and certain movements may not be as coordinated. The reduction in functional capability can lead to falls and accidental injuries. A program of regular exercise is generally useful to offset such potentially harmful changes.

There is a gradual progressive loss of skeletal muscle mass due to atrophy of muscle cells. Many of the atrophied muscle cells are replaced by fat and, eventually, by collagenous fibers.

Exercise and the Older Individual

Aerobic activities such as calisthenics, rapid walking, jogging, dancing, and hiking increase flexibility and overall endurance or aerobic power, but not strength. Older persons can increase their general physical fitness, particularly heart and lung fitness, with regular aerobic exercise. In many cases, the improvements exceed that seen in younger adults, and the results are that many older persons who regularly participate in endurance exercise are more physically fit than their sedentary middle-aged counterparts. Aerobic activities cause few injuries and cause fewer major adverse health consequences. Regular participation in such activities for a period of time increases overall fitness dramatically.

Weight training or other strength training can improve older person's strength and overall ability to function. Strength or resistance training increases the size and strength of muscles without improving endurance. Even octogenarians respond well to resistance training. Their muscles grow in size and strength much as do those of younger people. Success is largely dependent upon the frequency, intensity, and duration of training.

Weight training offers a number of benefits to older persons' health, including weight loss. Exercise can also be used to reduce the risk and complications of specific health problems such as coronary heart disease, high blood pressure, colon cancer, diabetes, arthritis, and osteoporosis. Regular exercise also helps to reduce the risk of falls and alleviates depression. The use of traditional weight machines is gradually spreading to long-term care facilities.

Mobility and Independence Aids

Persons who experience difficulty in performing exercises due to limitations in movement, can more conveniently engage in swimming as a means of exercise. A mini-pool that is four meters long and two meters wide can be installed in a room of the home, the garage, or in the office. This pool is equipped with a motorized paddle-wheel that creates a constant artificial current. The swimmer moves against the current or wave either by remaining in the same spot or by swimming the short pool length. The force of the current can be regulated through a control panel. This system allows the exerciser to move against the flow of water or to exercise by moving only a few meters or actually remaining stationary. The swimmer has the sensation of the water coming toward him or her as a wave in the sea. The small size of the pool makes it possible to install in the home or office.

With regard to prosthetic devices, the Seattle Foot (TM) is probably one of the most advanced simulators of human function. It is an artificial foot intended to be attached to a below-knee or above-knee prosthesis. The prosthetic foot contains a plastic keel within a cosmetic, anatomically detailed foam foot. This incredibly lifelike foot is designed so that the amputee can even wear sandals and thongs. The spring keel stores and releases energy as an amputee applies and removes force. In this manner, natural shock absorption and forward thrust are provided to the prosthetic leg. This allows activities such as walking, running, or jumping to be performed. Different keel spring rates are available to tailor the prosthesis to the individual. The Seattle Foot offers great promise to amputees. This intervention even allows persons to engage in sports activities, such as basketball.

Mobility adds reassurance to the individual. For patients with Alzheimer's disease and related problems, radioemitting devices may be worn to facilitate locating or finding these individuals when they are walking about the facility or the grounds for exercise. In a similar vein, telephone devices that dial automatically by squeezing may be used.

Personal emergency response systems such as Lifeline are now in use with increasing frequency. Lifeline is a personal emergency response system that allows an individual to press a small personal help button. This help button is worn on a chain around the neck or on a wrist strap. When pressed, the help button can link the individual to the Emergency Medical System, if needed. This allows increased independence and security for these individuals. This also leads to maintaining a continuation of personal life-style which can include independent movement and exercise.

Major technological advances have been made in the diagnosis, treatment, and aides to mobility regarding aging in general and podiatric gerontology in particular. Positive effects of technology have included the improved physical fitness, decreased mortality, improved home health care delivery, increased leisure, and the possibility of second or multiple careers for persons as they age. Robotics are becoming increasingly important in tasks such as ambulation, housekeeping, physical therapy, surveillance, and mental stimulation.

Ambulation Aids for the Elderly

Ambulation is a functional activity for which most physically impaired elderly patients must be carefully prepared. Those with lower extremity weakness or other impairment frequently benefit from walkers, canes, crutches, and wheelchairs. These devices, however, might not help–and may even be harmful–if they are given to persons physically incapable of using them or untrained in their proper use.

To determine whether a person will be able to use a device, it is important to evaluate the person's general condition and specific gait disability. It is futile to expect an individual to ambulate with crutches, cane, or walker if he or she lacks sufficient strength to do so. Muscle strength must be evaluated with particular ambulation needs in mind. People should be instructed never to use crutches, canes, walkers, or other such devices while in bare feet or loose slippers.

As with other ambulation aids, people must be trained to operate a wheelchair properly and safely. In addition, both the older person and the family must be cautioned about prolonged sitting and the possible dangers of decubiti and flexion contracture of the knees and hips.

REFERENCES

Andrews, G. R. (Ed). (1998). Ageing beyond 2000: One world one future. *Australian Journal on Aging, 17*(1), Supplement.

Butler, R. N., & Brody, J. A. (Eds.). (1995). *Delaying the Onset of Late-Life Dysfunction.* New York: Springer.

Chop, W. C., & Robnett, R. H. (1999). *Gerontology for the Health Care Professional.* Philadelphia: F.A. Davis.

Harris, R. (Ed.). (1983). *Medical devices and instrumentation for the elderly.* Arlington, VA: Association for the Advancement of Medical Instrumentation.

Lesnoff-Caravaglia, G. (Ed.). (1987). *Aging in a Technological Society.* New York: Human Sciences Press.

Lesnoff-Caravaglia, G. (Ed.). (1988). *Handbook of Applied Gerontology.* New York: Human Sciences Press.

Mann, W. C., Hurran, D., & Tomita, M. (1995). Assistive devices used by home-based elderly persons with arthritis. *The American Journal of Occupational Therapy, 49*(8), 810-819.

Oran, J. J. (1997). *Caring for the Fourth Age.* London: Armelle.

Rowe, J. W., & Kahn, R. (1998). *Successful Aging.* New York: Pantheon.

Spence, A. P. (1995). *Biology of Human Aging* (2nd ed.). Englewood Cliffs, NJ: Prentice-Hall.

Technology and Aging in America. (1985). TOA-BA-264. Washington, DC: U.S. Congress, Office of Technology Assessment.

Chapter 4

THE NERVOUS SYSTEM

The nervous system is composed of three types of organs: the brain, the spinal cord, and nerves. Internal communication among cells of the body is conducted by two body systems: the nervous system and the endocrine system.

The nervous system controls body movements through the contraction and relaxation of skeletal muscles and smooth muscles. Sensory information both from outside and inside the body is related to the nervous system, which it then processes and stores. Receptors in the nervous system link it to the special senses of vision, hearing, touch, taste, and smell.

The nervous system is also involved in activities that produce conscious remembering, thinking, interpretation, emotions, and personality traits. All of these higher-level functions take place in the brain. Changes in the nervous system due to senescence can slow the processing of information by the system and affect a person's memory and ability to accumulate and apply new information. The aging of the nervous system can be fraught with problems for the older individual.

As people age, there is a gradual loss of nerve cells. Since nerve cells are not replaced, an inevitable reduction in nervous tissue occurs. The effect of such losses varies among individuals and is largely dependent on the site. Since many more nerve cells are present than are requisite for the functioning of the nervous system, such losses may not become problematic until advanced old age.

As the brain ages, it becomes an increasingly finely balanced system. Although the aged brain has a capacity to compensate for damage and to repair itself, the process is limited. The brain has a large reserve capacity through a surplus of neurons and synapses. Depending upon the extent of neuron loss, brain functioning may not be affected. In fact, there is some indication that new nerve cell connections and new synapses may be formed to effectively compensate for those lost and to possibly even create new ones. The process of learning involves the formation of new synapses. Since learning continues throughout the life-span, this means that intellectual ability does not necessarily decline with age.

In general, highly educated people tend to retain their intellectual abilities longer than those who are not as well educated. Furthermore, people with high intelligence tend to live longer than those less well gifted.

The process of consciously remembering information is referred to as memory. Memory is also affected by age. There are at least three broad types of memory: short-term memory that retains information for only several seconds or minutes; intermediate memory that can last for several hours; and long-term memory that requires several hours or days to develop but can last a lifetime. Long-term memory seems to be less affected by age than is short-term memory. In fact, long-term memory seems to appreciably increase in older persons. Persons may have difficulty in remembering what they had for breakfast, but can relate with great detail events that occurred in their childhood.

Aging causes a decline in short-term memory in most people. The rate of decline varies highly between individuals. This may be due in part to differences in the rate of age changes within the nervous system, but it can be caused by other factors as well. Such factors include differences in general health, diet, presence of particular diseases, habitual levels of mental activity, motivation, economic conditions, psychological well-being, and socialization patterns. Such decline, however, since it is gradual and slow, allows for the development of compensatory strategies.

Memory retention does not show appreciable decline among persons endowed with higher intelligence. This also seems to be true of older persons who remain in the workplace or maintain active intellectual interests following retirement. Also, people who engage in social activities with family, friends, or by volunteering do not seem to suffer from memory deterioration. This could be related to the higher earning capabilities of such people and their consequent better standards of living and health care.

Changes in the brain itself as a result of aging occur primarily in the neurons of the hippocampus which is involved in functions such as memory. Neurofibrillary tangles and neuritic plaques begin to appear. A neurofibrillary tangle is composed of large groupings of fibrils or microtubules that develop in some neurons. Such clusters or tangles have been found only in the brains of human beings. They increase in number as persons continue to age, and are present in virtually all persons over the age of 80.

The significance of the presence of neuritic plaques and neurofibrillary tangles in aging brains is not well understood. Small numbers have been found in older persons who function well in old age, as well as in the brains of people who suffer from mental health problems. There appears to be a relationship between the number of plaques and tangles and the level of mental impairment. Plaques and tangles are present in significant numbers in brains of persons afflicted with Parkinson's disease, Down syndrome, and Alzheimer's disease.

Dysfunctions

Decreased Reflex Responses

As persons age, there is an alteration with respect to reflex responses. There is a gradual decrease in such responses and an absence of jerk reflexes of the ankle, biceps muscles, triceps muscles and the knee. Such changes may begin to be manifest by the age of 70, but, by the age of 90, such jerk reflexes seem to have been lost.

Sleep

The aging process appears to affect the length, distribution, and pattern of sleep. Sleep disorders or expressed dissatisfaction with the quality or quantity of sleep are common complaints in old age.

More difficulty is experienced in falling asleep, more time is needed to fall asleep, there are frequent awakenings during the night, and, once awakened, it takes longer to return to sleep. Some causative factors for such changes include the presence of pain, indigestion, use of medications, anxiety, nocturia, along with respiratory or circulatory problems. The increase in awakenings is greater in men than in women.

Changes occur in the type of sleep. Sleep is divided into two types: rapid-eye-movement (REM) sleep and nonrapid-eye-movement

(NREM). They are designated as such because of the eye movements that occur during each period. During NREM sleep, sleep becomes progressively deeper with brain activity slowing and regularizing. This is followed by REM sleep during which dreaming occurs. REM sleep and NREM sleep alternate during much of the sleep cycle, with periods of REM sleep occurring about every 80 to 100 minutes. During REM sleep, recordings of brain activity resemble those of an alert, awake brain. In contrast, during NREM sleep, brain recordings show lower frequency waves and the respiratory rate, heart rate, and blood pressure are generally below waking levels. It has been suggested that physiological recuperation occurs during deep NREM sleep.

Although the time spent sleeping changes little with age, significant alteration in sleep patterns often occur. Sleep becomes more shallow and is less sound and efficient. For example, the ratio between REM sleep and slow-wave sleep gradually changes with age, resulting in fewer episodes of deep sleep. Older people also complain of problems such as difficulty falling asleep, awakening frequently during the night, awakening early in the morning, and a feeling of fatigue—even after a night's sleep. One of the most frequent complaints, voiced by about 40 percent of the elderly, is their inability to sleep long enough or peacefully enough to feel rested. This problem is referred to as insomnia.

An area of the brain stem known as the reticular activating system is thought to control brain alertness. Changes in sleep patterns with aging may be related in part to alterations in the reticular activating system. If the system maintains the brain in an alert state, a person cannot sleep. Thus, most medications that induce sleep do so by depressing the reticular activating system. Other factors are also thought to contribute to the high incidence of insomnia in the elderly, including frequent daytime naps, anxiety, and depression.

The effects of age-related changes in sleep include a reduction in the quality of sleep. These effects probably explain why more people feel sleepy during the day as they get older. However, this is not a normal part of aging. It is difficult to determine how much or which of the changes in sleep are due to aging of the brain and which are due to other age-related factors, such as having diseases, taking more medication, being past menopause, having different daily routines because of retirement, having more freedom for daytime napping, and experiencing altered social situations such as death of a spouse or a move to a different home or institution.

Dementia

Dementia is a broad category of diseases which generally presents with a decline in memory and often with major deficits in one or more additional areas of mental functioning. While the number and rate of cases of dementia are increasing, there has been a tendency to overestimate the incidence of dementia among the old and to underestimate that of depression.

People over 65 years of age are the fastest growing segment of the American population. Vitally important to the quality of life is the maintenance of cognitive function. Though decline may occur, age alone need not result in the loss of such function. While some succumb to disease and deterioration, certain individuals manage to "age successfully," maintaining high levels of intellectual functionality throughout life. Very few cases occur in people below age 60.

Age-related dementia nominally results in the loss of cognitive function, affecting, in particular, the ability to recall events. Functions that are often reduced include speaking, reading, writing, solving problems, and performing simple voluntary tasks. Dementia can also cause behavioral disturbances, as well as a wide range of changes that indicate mental deterioration.

It has been estimated that over 30 percent of the population over the age of 85 experience severe dementia. As life expectancy continues to increase, the prevalence of severe dementia will probably rise in the future. Large numbers of nursing home residents currently suffer from some form of dementia.

There are more than 60 different types of dementia. Some forms of dementia are caused by such things as anemia, nutritional deficiencies, medications, and depression. These forms are reversible when appropriate treatment is provided. Another group in which brain deterioration has markedly advanced are considered as irreversible. Atherosclerosis of the blood vessels of the brain or reduced blood supply is largely responsible for the irreversible forms of dementia. The ischemia (deficiency of blood) can be of short duration and not lead necessarily to mental or functional impairment or to brain deterioration. It can, however, be conducive to vertigo, falls, and accidents.

Alzheimer's Disease

Dementia caused by Alzheimer's disease is also known as senile dementia of the Alzheimer's type (SDAT). While Alzheimer's Disease is very rare in persons under the age of 65, it affects one person in 10 over the age of 65. It is found in approximately 15 percent of the 65-74 year-old population, and rises to over 45 percent in the 85+ population. Alzheimer disease is the most frequent cause of institutionalization for long-term care, and accounts for an estimated 30 to 50 percent of those in nursing homes. Alzheimer's disease is often misdiagnosed; 8 to 23 percent of those said to have this disease may actually be suffering from depression or other treatable disorders.

Alzheimer's disease is an organic brain disease named after the German physician, Alios Alzheimer, who first described it in 1906. Alzheimer's disease causes progressive loss of mental functions over a period of years. Its clinical progression is usually divided into three stages:

1. There is a decrease in short-term memory and attention. Difficulties in speech and word-finding; loss of the ability to "think through" complex actions or to interpret complex stimuli, and disorientation to time and place. Memory function declines to such an extent that affected individuals have difficulty in performing ordinary daily activities such as preparing food, dressing, and shopping. The first signs noted can, however, vary greatly from person to person.

2. This is followed by worsening cognitive deterioration and personality changes, often including irritability, and severe disorientation as to time and place. The patient's speech often remains fluent and grammatical, but the content of what is said is often inappropriate or disconnected from reality.

3. Finally, the patient shows complete loss of intellectual abilities, leading to a state of vegetation. This includes the inability to speak or to recognize even close relatives, and complete loss of "world knowledge." Confusion occurs easily and frequently, and many patients wander away from home and become lost. More advanced effects may include paranoia, hostility, aggressiveness and outburst of anger. The nervous system seems to forget how to stimulate muscles so that walking, eating, and other voluntary motions dwindle and finally cease. The final result of Alzheimer's disease is death.

There is great variation in the duration of the illness and its rate of progression. Younger patients tend to have more severe cases which progress more rapidly. Alzheimer's disease can last from a few years to a few decades. There are no effective means of prevention. This disorder is slightly more common in females than in males.

Alzheimer's Disease compromises the ability to learn and to recall information and the ability to control and to execute meaningful changes in behavior. Early in the course of the disease, patients cannot recall names or places recently experienced. As the disease progresses, the individual develops an inability to control behavior and may display increased aggressiveness, wandering, and agitation. The ability to execute meaningful changes in behavior is lost. The disease selectively attacks the most plastic among the brain's centers, striking first the malleable circuits engaged in learning and memory, then undermines the more stable functions responsible for higher cognition and behavioral control, finally compromising the personality itself. An autopsy is required to confirm a diagnosis of Alzheimer's disease.

One of the serious consequences of this disease is that it frequently involves the entire family in caregiving roles. When the caregiver is the spouse or a daughter, the life of this individual is often devoted to caring for the Alzheimer's patient. The unfortunate aspect to Alzheimer's Disease is that the individual is gradually lost to the family and even to him or herself, even though physically present.

Heredity seems to play a role in the transmission of Alzheimer's disease. It is usually transmitted from female to female, and can be present in 3 or 4 generations of the same family. Not only direct descendants, but nieces and cousins have been affected. From 30 percent to 50 percent of the cases appear to be inherited.

Recent research has resulted in the isolation of two genetic markers on chromosome 21 that may point to the gene responsible for the condition. Also, a gene that is responsible for the formation of the neuritic plaques was identified on chromosome 21. The linkage of stress and nutrition as potential causative factors has also engaged the attention of researchers.

One of the major consequences of the onset of Alzheimer's disease is the progressive loss of intellectual competence. Loss of judgment, memory, and many other intellectual skills make it increasingly difficult for the person to function independently. Such alterations in functioning place increasing burdens upon caregivers who ultimately must take responsibility not only for the physical care, but for the behavioral control as well. Chemical and physical changes in the brain can account for some of the memory deficits in Alzheimer's disease and for benign forgetfulness of some older persons.

Moderate declines in intellectual competence in well-functioning older persons may simply result from disuse. Decline in intellectual abilities is not characteristic of all persons as they age. Individual differences are heightened by different life-styles. The maintenance or decline of cognitive functions can be significantly affected by life-style factors. Although not a universal fact, substantial decline in intellectual competence may become evident in the mid-80s to early 90s and is frequently linked to disease states. Diminishment in intellectual functioning can become apparent prior to death and is known as "terminal drop."

Unfavorable environments and maladaptive life-styles may be responsible for both increased risk for cardiovascular disease and for intellectual decline. The lack of stimulating environments, disengaged life-styles, inflexible attitudes, and lack of supportive interpersonal networks may all contribute to intellectual decline. The intellectual competence of older persons can be increased by suitable training and alteration of environmental conditions.

Non-Alzheimer Dementias

Some forms of dementia include cognitive and behavioral changes which are often mistaken for Alzheimer's disease. Such changes do not generally follow a progressive pattern. Changes can be sudden in nature, but remain constant for long periods of time. Some persons may have memory problems, but the ability to function within a normal range is unimpaired.

Dementia caused by circulatory disease is referred to as multi-infarct dementia. Nearly 30 percent of all dementia cases fall under this heading. In this condition, decreased periods of blood flow to the brain alternate with periods of adequate blood flow. Such discontinuity results in ministrokes or transient ischemic attacks (TIAs). The repetition of ministrokes may damage small areas of the brain. The damage, however, may be so slight that the person is not aware of the occurrence. Cells in the damaged regions of the brain do die, however, and degeneration of the areas is the result of such infarcts. A long history of such ministrokes can lead to Alzheimer's-like symptoms, memory loss, and absent-minded behavior.

Parkinson's Disease

Parkinson's disease refers to a clinical condition characterized by muscular rigidity and a rhythmic tremor. It is a leading disease of the nervous system among older persons. It is chronic with symptoms slowly progressing over an extended period of time that can reach 15 to 20 years. Symptoms are usually noted at approximately age 50. The highest rate of incidence occurs at approximately the age of 75. This condition is found more commonly in men than in women. Many persons afflicted with this disease eventually develop Alzheimer's disease. For this reason, Parkinson's disease is described as a form of dementia. Afflicted persons also experience deep depression, anxiety attacks, and suicidal ideation. As symptoms increase in severity over the years, the person may continue to be mentally sound and alert.

Parkinson's disease has essentially three basic components: rigidity, tremors, and diminished spontaneous movements. Spontaneous movements, such as swinging of the arms when walking, changing positions and crossing legs while sitting down, are diminished or absent. Akinesia and rigidity are probably responsible for mask-like facies, monotonous speech, and slowness of movement. The useless contractions of skeletal muscles cause not only muscle rigidity but tremors. The tremors, which are present at rest, become less when movement is initiated. They are absent during periods of sleep.

Persons with Parkinson's disease have a characteristic gait. The general posture is that of flexion: the knees are slightly flexed and the trunk appears flexed and bent forward; the elbows and wrists are also flexed. They may take short shuffling steps and tend to lean forward. Although the initiation of the first few steps is slow, the person appears as if glued to the floor, then starts to walk faster and faster. If suddenly asked to stop and turn around, the person may be unable to do so. Persons with Parkinson's disease are particularly at risk of falling. They cannot take avoiding actions to stop the fall or at least to reduce its impact.

A stooped posture is characteristic of this disease, with a tendency for the head to fall forward. Speech is slow and monotonous, and there may be some drooling from the mouth and watering of the eyes. Handwriting deteriorates, and there is often loss of facial expression. Many persons experience great frustration as these losses progress.

As control of muscle contraction diminishes further, the patient may find it impossible to complete a motion once it has been started. A person who is walking may suddenly stop in the middle of taking a step. Muscle contractions for swallowing and breathing also weaken and slow. Declining muscle control and muscle activity causes drooling. Severe disability can be delayed for many years.

The detection of early cases may sometimes be difficult, and no definite cause has been identified. Some theories posit stress as a possible cause and extend stress to include stressful experiences at birth, such as breech births. Although the cause is unknown, it is thought to be a bio-chemical imbalance in the brain. This occurs when cells of the basal ganglia fail to properly metabolize the neurotransmitter dopamine. One treatment is the administration of L-dopa, which is a precursor of dopamine. L-dopa is able to cross the blood-brain barrier and enter the brain cells, where it is converted into dopamine. L-dopa diminishes muscle rigidity and tremors. It improves posture and speech, but has little effect on altering the mask-like facial appearance.

Surgical transplantation of tissue from an adrenal gland into the brain continues to show promising results. This is particularly the case when the intervention is made in the early stages of the disease and on a younger patient. The use of gland tissue from fetuses initially prompted extensive ethical controversy. The tissue can also be extracted from the afflicted individual.

Cerebrovascular Accident

Cerebrovascular accident (CVA) or stroke originates as a disease of the cardiovascular system. Strokes are the third leading cause of death among people over the age of 65. The death rates from strokes and heart disease have steadily declined due to better prevention of atherosclerosis and better diagnosis and treatment of strokes and heart disease.

A stroke occurs when blood flow to and through the brain is disrupted. Because of the sudden and devastating effects on the brain, the victim appears to have been struck with a heavy blow, and thus the term "stroke" was adopted. Since strokes affect the brain and are usually caused by abnormalities in the blood vessels, such as a buildup of fatty deposits or a blood clot, or in the heart, they are also referred to as cerebrovascular accidents (CVAs).

Many people who have a stroke survive. The neurological effects of a stroke vary, depending on the side and extent of brain damage.

Large strokes may cause paralysis or dementia. The death rates due to stroke increase substantially in individuals over the age of 65. Many survivors loose the capacity to walk, to speak, and to read. Many experience confused mental states affecting memory and the capability to think clearly. Severe depression is a common aftermath.

Physical symptoms produced by a stroke generally appear on the opposite side of the body from the side of the brain in which the lesion occurred. This is caused by the fact that most of the nerve tracts connecting the brain and spinal cord cross. Those who survive are often left with serious lifelong disabilities.

Strokes occur more frequently in men than in women. Their incidence is significantly higher in the Black population than in the White population. This is the case in both men and women. Life-style factors are often contributing factors.

The debilities left in the wake of a stroke often cause the individual to feel depressed. Changes in performance abilities have an effect upon self-esteem and personal identity. Alterations in the capability to write or the length of time it may require, for example, hold great ramifications in terms of whether or not the person will sustain correspondence or will withdraw. It is often difficult to dictate personal correspondence to another individual, and the dependency may weigh heavily upon the person. Also, the manner in which one signs his or her name is a personal expression of self. It is an expression of one's own individuality. People dot their i's or write their names in idiosyncratic ways that they feel to be original. Experiencing a stroke may alter many of these writing behaviors. Not being able to sign one's own name can be traumatic.

Microsurgery and New Nerve Pathways

Microsurgery which is used primarily in reconstructive surgery has been utilized to develop new pathways for severed nerves. It functions very much like a coronary bypass in that once the ordinary pathway is no longer usable, a new one is initiated to continue nerve function. Just as it has become possible to attach severed limbs and to have them function, it is now possible to mend severed nerves and to allow them to function once again. Spinal cord lesions can be repaired through the introduction of such new pathways to allow paraplegics and persons with nerve damage to recover their mobility. The peripheral nervous system is utilized in resolving spinal cord dysfunctions, with the brain adapting to this new pattern. The nervous system "bypass" also creates new cerebral circuits which activate leg muscle movements. For older individuals, nerve damage can thus be repaired and limb functions can be improved.

Rehabilitation of Senile Dementia Patients

Patients with severe brain damage can be retrained so that impaired cognitive processes are reacquired through different routes, using healthy brain tissue. Electronic television games have a compelling, almost addictive, attraction for many people. It appears likely that this would apply to elderly people suffering from senile dementia. Participation in games can help develop alertness and lengthen attention span.

Social or Psychosocial Therapies

The role of social or psychosocial therapies is to optimize or maximize the adaptive capacity of the older individual by providing assistance and support where necessary, and gradually and appropriately withdrawing those supports in order to help the person retain control over his or her own life to the greatest extent possible. Such supports may be personal, cognitive, emotive, or insightful. They may be administered through the traditional or innovative psychological or social psychological therapies; they may be identified as educational or social rather than therapeutic.

The traditional mental health strategy has been related to the detection and treatment of illness, a sickness-oriented rather than a prevention health-oriented perspective. The focus should properly be on maximizing the potential of the older person in his or her environment.

Biological systems in aging are almost all downward systems. On the other hand, the aging process also carries with it the opportunity for increased personal growth. Personal historical perspectives, when coupled with the experiences of a life long-lived, provide a valuable framework from which to determine individual choice and to assess societal behaviors. Such seasoned judgment has long gone under the heading of wisdom.

Nevertheless, many older persons experience an appreciable loss of mastery over the environment. Social losses usually increase after the age of 70. Such losses include the death of friends or relatives, sensory losses, loss of control over one's body, and loss of decisionmaking powers. Social environmental forces shape life in ways which may alleviate or exacerbate physical and mental health and their interrelationship. Life events can promote both diseases of the mind and body. The future role of mental health providers may well be to prepare and to educate aging persons to the complexity of factors which determine healthy mental functioning in advanced old age.

Changes in demography and in the social construct of the environment in the future, due to the baby-boomers, will add yet another dimension to the responsibilities of health and social services. The broader society needs to be made aware of the needs and stresses that increasing numbers of older persons will face. Society and mental health professionals need to prepare and to plan for an older population that will experience a shift in roles from programmed activity to leisure or voluntary activity, to a new career, to retraining, and to a variety of options with respect to life-styles and living environments.

It is important that sufficient support systems are available to assist persons to make such significant shifts which range from changes in cognitive capacity to changes in economic status. Society must be prepared as to what to expect of the older population and what it needs. The development of support groups that focus on significant losses such as widowhood or profound life-style changes may be required, in addition to the intensified interventions by health or social service providers.

Viewing the whole person against the background of his or her personal environment may be more helpful in arriving at an assessment of the older person's mental health care needs, the role of life events, and the ensuing stresses that evolve. It is not age or disease alone that affect the mental health status and functioning of older individuals.

REFERENCES

Andrews, G. R. (Ed). (1998). Ageing beyond 2000: One world one future. *Australian Journal on Aging, 17* (1), Supplement.

Butler, R. N. & Brody, J. A. (Eds.). (1995). *Delaying the Onset of Late-Life Dysfunction.* New York: Springer.

DiGiovanna, A. G. (1994). *Human Aging.* New York: McGraw-Hill.

Harris, R., (Ed.). (1983). *Medical devices and instrumentation for the elderly.* Arlington, VA: Association for the Advancement of Medical Instrumentation.

Kart, C. S. (1997). *The Realities of Aging.* Boston: Allyn & Bacon.

Kart, C. S., Metress, E. K., & Metress, S. P. (1992). *Human Aging and Chronic Disease.* Boston: Bartlett & Jones.

Lesnoff-Caravaglia, G. (Ed.). (1987). *Aging in a Technological Society.* New York: Human Sciences Press.

Lesnoff-Caravaglia, G. (Ed.). (1988). *Handbook of Applied Gerontology.* New York: Human Sciences Press.

Mann, W. C., Hurren, D., & Tomita, M. (1995). Assistive devices used by home-based elderly persons with arthritis. *The American Journal of Occupational Therapy, 49* (8), 810-819.

Oram, J. J. (1997). *Caring for the Fourth Age.* London: Armelle.

Rowe, J.W., & Kahn, R. (1998). *Successful Aging.* New York: Pantheon.

Spence, A.P. (1995). *Biology of Human Aging* (2nd. ed.). Englewood Cliffs, NJ: Prentice-Hall.

Technology and Aging in America. (1985). TOA-BA-264. Washington, DC: U.S. Congress, Office of Technology Assessment.

contraction~ systole
relaxation~ diastole

Chapter 5

THE CIRCULATORY SYSTEM

The circulatory system contains several very different components and is the system that most directly affects the total functioning of the body. The supplying of the body with nutrients and the carrying off of waste deposits is essential to body maintenance, and the heart (myocardium) is the key to its functioning. The lymphatic system assists in this process through its filtering processes and the deneutralizing of toxins carried out by organs such as the liver, tonsils, and the spleen. This constant progress throughout the body is carried on by the propelling of the blood through the veins and arteries by the rhythmic beating of the heart.

There are four chambers to the heart, and the heart has two rhythms, one of contraction (systole) and of relaxation (diastole). This regular beat forms the pulse which is a significant vital sign for determining proper cardiovascular functioning. The veins and the arteries are the principal pathways for the movement of blood to and from the heart. Arteries have thicker walls and experience the greatest propulsion of blood against their walls.

For the cells of the body to survive, to grow, and to function properly, they must receive a constant supply of oxygen and various nutrients. They must also be able to dispose of waste products in an expeditious manner. The structures of the circulatory system are particularly well designed to carry out such activities.

The importance of the circulatory system is intensified in old age. Diseases of the circulatory system become increasingly a problem as they significantly affect all bodily systems. The major causes of death in the United States and many developed countries is from diseases of the heart and the blood vessels. The two primary causes of death, heart disease and stroke, are both the result of circulatory system dys-

2 main causes of death: 1. h. disease
                        2. stroke

function. Those who survive the onslaught of such diseases can be left with a variety of disabilities. Some persons may experience a total change in life-style, including abandonment of work roles and recreational pursuits. Interpersonal relationships can be affected. Dependency becomes a significant factor, and transfer from life in the community to an institutional setting may become a reality for more severely disabled persons. Home health care can provide assistance in the private home setting, but such services are frequently unavailable or too costly for many older individuals.

The circulatory system includes both the cardiovascular and lymphatic systems. The heart and blood vessels comprise the cardiovascular system. Blood is propelled by the rhythmic contractions of the heart, essentially a pump, through the blood vessels. This is a closed system that forms a circular path or round trip throughout the body. Blood travels through the heart into arteries and veins, and then back to the heart. The lymphatic system includes the lymphatic vessels and the lymphoid organs, such as the tonsils, thymus, spleen, lymph nodes, and lymphoid nodules.

The aging changes that occur in the heart generally do not affect its functioning sufficiently well to sustain the reduced level of activity generally engaged in by older persons. Diseases that interfere or disrupt the blood flow through the coronary arteries to the heart muscle can seriously reduce the heart's capacity to maintain normal activities.

It is quite likely that disease and life-style may have a greater influence on cardiovascular function than does aging. Abuse of alcohol, tobacco products, obesity, improper general diet, lack of exercise, and stress compromise the effectiveness of the cardiovascular system. Such life-style factors when prevalent throughout the life span manifest their consequences in old age. Not only the diseases that people contract, but the medications used to treat these diseases can ultimately affect the cardiovascular system.

Dysfunctions

Many of the dysfunctions that occur in the circulatory system do not originate in old age. Many are initiated at much younger ages, and, since people are living longer, such problems have time to mature and to develop and only manifest themselves when people grow old. Such dysfunctions increase in number as persons age, and their presence often as chronic disorders serve to seriously compromise health. The most obvious contributing factors are those of life-style.

Atherosclerosis and Arteriosclerosis

Atherosclerosis is the disease that prevents the coronary arteries from supplying adequate blood flow to the heart. The formation of and enlargement of material called "plaque" in the walls of the arteries causes the coronary arteries to become narrower and thus reduces blood flow. It also stiffens arteries, much like old bicycle tires, reducing their ability to dilate when more oxygen is needed by the heart muscle. Plaques can also contribute to the formation of clots which can completely prevent blood flow. When blood flow to the body drops, all the organs perform less well. The brain, kidneys, lungs, and heart are especially in danger because these organs require a high level of blood flow. A low level of oxygen can lead to the death of the heart muscle, resulting in a myocardial infarction (heart attack).

As the life expectancy of the general population increases, more people can be expected to develop atherosclerotic occlusive disease. Although the cause of atherosclerosis is not known, its frequent association with the degenerative aging process is widely accepted. Age itself is not a contraindication to surgical treatment of this disease in selected cases. When one considers the potential risk of operation versus the potential gain, the patient's physiologic age as well as associated diseases should be evaluated. Many elderly patients have associated cardiac, pulmonary, or renal diseases. Yet, in the properly selected elderly patient, careful preoperative preparation can be helpful in the successful outcome of a major operation such as peripheral vascular surgery.

In advanced cases of atherosclerosis, plaques can become hardened by the deposition of calcium, and fibrous tissue may collect in the arterial walls. Such a condition can lead to arteriosclerosis, or hardening of the arteries. The changes in the arterial walls with arteriosclerosis greatly reduce their elasticity. As a result, the vessels are less able to respond to the blood pressure changes that occur as the heart contracts and relaxes. Weakened areas of the vessel wall may also dilate to form a bubble-like aneurysm that could easily rupture when blood pressure reaches higher levels.

While it is not totally clear exactly how plaque forms, a variety of interventions have been employed. One such preventive method indicates that lowering low-density lipoprotein levels and raising high-density lipoprotein levels will lower blood cholesterol. This could serve to prevent cerebrovascular disease. Most of the factors contributing to the development of atherosclerosis have been identified, and many of them can be avoided or reduced. Many of these factors are related to life-style and include simple measures such as stopping smoking, drinking less coffee, and lowering blood pressure.

Cardiovascular diseases in combination with other major diseases can present serious health problems. Persons suffering from diabetes, for example, may experience reduced blood flow to the extremities which can lead to the development of gangrene and limb amputation. Amputees are frequently older persons, and the clientele of rehabilitation centers increasingly include the elderly.

Hypertension

Hypertension, or high blood pressure, is a problem of all age groups, but it is found more commonly among older persons. It is also known as the silent killer. In older persons, hypertension is generally linked to atherosclerosis and arteriosclerosis. Blood pressure represents the force exerted by blood flowing against vessel walls created by the pumping action of the heart. Elevated blood pressure is potentially serious because it can contribute to heart attack, heart failure, stroke, renal failure, or rupture of blood vessels.

Elevated blood pressure can often be lowered and maintained at more normal levels through modifications of diet or with various medications. A reduction in the use of sodium (salt) or the consumption of salty foods is an important preventive measure.

High blood pressure is not an inevitable consequence of aging. Life-style contributes more to the development of hypertension and heart disease than does the process of aging. Harmful life-style factors include lack of exercise, obesity, excessive alcohol consumption, excessive intake of salt, and smoking. Drinking exorbitant amounts of coffee is often added to the list.

It is possible for persons to experience minor heart attacks and to not realize exactly what has occurred. Some persons can have as many as three or four small such attacks and attribute their discomfort to indigestion or other ailments. The system is weakened because of these episodes, and when a stronger attack occurs, it can result in death.

Coronary Artery Disease

Coronary artery disease results when insufficient blood flows through the coronary arteries to the heart muscle. Ischemic heart disease results when tissue does not receive a supply of blood sufficient to maintain its cells. The reduced blood flow is due to a narrowing or constriction of the coronary arteries caused by plaque formation.

Such decreases in coronary artery blood flow in old age increase the likelihood of coronary artery disease. In fact, it is the major cause of heart problems and death among the elderly. There is also an increased incidence of coronary artery disease among postmenopausal women which may be caused by sudden increases in blood cholesterol levels.

The most frequent cause of diminished coronary blood flow is the development of plaques in the lining of the vessels. Such plaques may grow in size and eventually form a thrombus. The clot or thrombus can break off and move to a smaller coronary artery, where it may completely occlude the vessel. Some sections of the heart may be immediately deprived of blood. A blood clot or thrombus that travels within a vessel to another area is called an embolus.

The symptoms that result from a sudden blockage of a coronary artery are what is called a heart attack. A blocked coronary artery can be treated through bypass surgery in which a portion of an artery from another region of the body is grafted to the coronary artery and used to direct blood around the blocked portion. Another treatment procedure involves the injection of chemicals to dissolve the clot to restore blood flow, while, at the same time, a small catheter with a miniature balloon on its tip is entered through the vessel to the location of the clot. The balloon is inflated which then compresses the clot and opens the vessel. This procedure is known as balloon angioplasty. Still another method is one by which laser beams transmitted through fine glass fibers within a catheter remove the clot.

Coronary heart disease has traditionally been considered a problem which predominantly affects men; its extent and poor prognosis in

↘leading cause of death for women.

women have only recently been identified. According to the Framingham Study, women are more likely than men to die after myocardial infarction; this is now also evident after coronary artery bypass graft surgery and coronary angioplasty. However, the prognosis is currently also influenced by access to coronary diagnostic procedures and treatments, which may in turn be affected by factors such as womens' and their doctors' decisions about diagnostic procedures and treatments, by the location of health care resources, and by society's perceptions of the importance of coronary heart disease in women.

Coronary heart disease is more dependent on age in women than in men; women are usually 10 years older than men when any coronary manifestations first appear, and myocardial infarction occurs as much as 20 years later. One in 8 or 9 American women aged 45-64 years has clinical evidence of coronary heart disease, and this increases to 1 in 3 in women older than 65 years. Coronary heart disease is the leading cause of death in women in the United States. With the aging of the population, more women than men now die of coronary heart disease each year in the United States.

A White postmenopausal woman in the United States is 10 times more likely to die of heart disease than of breast cancer. Most women, however, do not understand the coronary threat. In many industrialized nations, it is now the major cause of death in postmenopausal women and a principal contributor to hospital admission and consultations with doctors.

The prevalence of risk factors is high in women of all racial and ethnic groups in the United States. American women aged 65 and over pay less attention to exercise and diet and use fewer other preventive health services than younger women. Risk factors are more prevalent in socioeconomically and educationally disadvantaged women; in the United States almost twice as many women as men aged 65 years of older are at the poverty level. The only risk factor more pronounced in younger women than in older women is smoking. Stopping smoking, however, benefits all persons, regardless of age.

Cholesterol concentrations continue to predict coronary risk in older women. Coronary heart disease is the major cause of death in postmenopausal women in many industrialized countries and will become epidemic in elderly women as the population ages unless preventive interventions across the life span are undertaken. Risk factors for coronary heart disease in older women must be evaluated and preventive measures instituted throughout a woman's lifetime. Also, mortality and morbidity after myocardial infarction and coronary revascularization procedures are greater in women than in men. Characteristics and treatments likely to be associated with better outcomes in older women need to be identified.

Physical inactivity is a highly prevalent and independent risk factor in women, although data are limited for elderly women. Exercise reduces coronary risk, even at older ages. Moderate leisuretime activity (30-45 minutes' walking three times weekly) reduces the risk of myocardial infarction by half.

Angina pectoris is the main initial and subsequent presenting symptom of coronary heart disease in women, while myocardial infarction and sudden death are the predominant presentations in men. Women with angina are likely to be older than men and to have hypotension, diabetes, and heart failure more commonly. Diabetes is a far greater risk factor for women than men. Women over 45 years of age are twice as likely as men to develop diabetes.

Women, on the whole, are not as aggressively treated with regard to coronary heart disease; they are half as likely to receive acute catheterization, coronary angioplasty, thrombolysis, or coronary artery bypass surgery.

Myocardial Infarction

Following an acute coronary artery blockage, blood flow ceases in the coronary vessels beyond the blockage. The area which, as a result, has either no blood flow or very little is subsequently damaged. This condition becomes what is known as a myocardial infarction or, more commonly, a heart attack. The presence of infarcted areas and the extent of the damage can be detected by an electrocardiogram (EKG).

Angina Pectoris

Short episodes of cardiac pain that result from progressive constriction of the coronary arteries is known as angina pectoris. The pain varies among individuals. The pain surfaces each time the heart has to contract more strenuously beyond that which can be supported by the restricted coronary blood flow. It has been described as sharp pressure, a dull ache, or as a form of constriction. People who have chronic angina pectoris feel the pain when they exercise or when they experience emotions that cause the heart rate to accelerate. The pain is usually described as being deep in the center of the chest. However, people do report feeling as if it were on the surface of the body, principally in the left arm and shoulder, the neck, and the side of the face. There are people, however, who have major heart attacks without experiencing angina pectoris.

Due to their reduced level of physical activity, there is a lower incidence of angina attacks in older persons. Treatment of angina generally involves the use of drugs that either dilate the arteries (e.g., nitroglycerin) or block the receptors that stimulate the sympathetic nervous system (e.g., beta blockers).

Congestive Heart Failure

Congestive heart failure or cardiac insufficiency is another disease that becomes more common and serious with age. Congestive heart failure is a condition in which the heart cannot pump enough blood to meet bodily needs. Actually, the condition itself is not a disease, but is more the result of other cardiovascular diseases that have so damaged the heart that it no longer functions adequately.

Because the heart cannot pump efficiently, blood collects in tissues. Edema (swelling) of the legs and ankles is common. When fluid backs up into the lungs, shortness of breath results, and people have difficulty breathing, particularly in supine positions. Congestive heart failure does not have a favorable prognosis. Drugs, however, that increase the contractile strength of the cardiac muscle and eliminate excess fluid from the body are helpful. Modification of diet, along with rest, is frequently recommended. Surgical interventions including repair of defective valves or other structural problems can also reduce the severity of heart failure.

In the presence of cardiac insufficiency the functioning of the entire body is compromised. Should problems arise in other organs, such as the kidneys or liver, these problems will be exacerbated by the heart condition. The heart is key to the smooth and efficient functioning of all systems. Muscular activity can be limited and participation in a variety of vocational or recreational activities may well be restricted.

Not only is there a reduction in the distribution of nutrients to the body, but the removal of waste products can be greatly slowed down. Foreign matter can linger or remain in regions of the body.

Arrhythmia

Irregular heartbeats can be the result of cardiovascular problems, or, in some people, can be an inherited characteristic. Persons who suffered from certain childhood disease such as rheumatic fever generally experience arrhythmia. In persons for whom this is a new phenomenon, it may indicate the presence of heart disease.

Technology and Interventions

The circulatory system can function efficiently and maintain appropriate blood flow that adequately supplies the needs of the body with respect to nutrients and oxygen even in advanced ages such as 90 or 100. What comprises the functioning of the system is the presence of diseases which frequently were initiated by unhealthy life-styles. People are very resistant to change and, even those habits which they realize are harmful, will be persisted in to the detriment of the health of the individual and, on occasion, the family's health. There are benefits to be derived from the cessation of smoking or altering the diet at the age of 80. The negative attitude which enforced the regarding of intervention and older persons as a futile effort, militated against recommending life-style changes or even researching their ultimate benefits. Since increases in life expectancy were undervalued or unexpected, persons over the age of 70 were regarded as rapidly approaching death and the overlooking of unhealthy life-styles was a form of patronizing kindness. At age 70, many persons can expect to live a minimum of an additional 15 years. Not informing older persons of the risks they incur because of life-style is a form of negligence. An essential ingredient in health care of the elderly is the educating of older persons.

Environmental factors continue to be an additional concern with regard to the maintenance of the equilibrium of the circulatory system. Unhealthy work environments can wreak havoc with a person's circulatory system which can result in serious debility in the later years of life or can shorten life expectancy. One example is black lung which affects miners and is the result of breathing in coal dust.

Some medical and surgical interventions are not indicated for older persons because their health is already compromised by other diseases from which they may be suffering. Bypass surgery, laser treatments, or angioplasty may not be recommended for some patients, but there are patients of advanced ages whose health can permit the use of more radical interventions. Ethical dilemmas with respect to the cost of such interventions and the appropriateness of their utilization continue to surface as the population continues to age and more people request such interventions.

Many of the interventions with respect to the circulatory system are commonly known, but simply not practiced. Educating people of all ages with regard to appropriate health care from birth to death can mean enhancing people's lives, making health care less costly, and extending the life expectancy.

Despite medical and surgical advances, congestive heart failure occurs with increasing frequency and remains a major source of morbidity and mortality, especially as the population ages.

Heart failure develops over time with two components. The first is a myocardium dysfunction due to an inadequate adaptive response to a work overload created either by primary damage or excess load, or loss of myocardium (acute myocardial infarction). The second component is congestive heart failure, resulting from reduced ventricular function with limited organ function, reduced exercise performance and sodium accumulation with edema. The process of aging alters the structure of the heart and contributes to primary cardiac dysfunction. The incidence of heart failure has increased progressively over the past three decades, and it now comprises a major source of morbidity and mortality in the American population, especially as the population ages. In patients over the age of 65, heart failure has now become the most common diagnostic related group category (DRG) for hospitalized patients. This increase in the incidence of heart failure has occurred despite major advances in the treatment of what has been thought to be primary etiological factors initiating the problem, namely hypertension, valvular disease, and ischemic heart disease. The passage of years allow primary abnormalities such as coronary atherosclerosis to play a progressively increasing role in the evolution of the disease.

Surgical Interventions

A healthy life-style and medical checkups are the principal ways to ensure a healthy cardiovascular system. However, when a cardiac problem is diagnosed, in addition to an appropriate diet and sufficient exercise, the use of drugs frequently is the next step. When such remedies are no longer effective, then surgical intervention is necessary.

If the problem involves cardiac insufficiency, new pathways can be used to furnish the obstructed area by using arteries from other areas, such as the stomach. This intervention is not without its problematic aspects, but it is one method for revitalizing the pumping action of the heart.

Another surgical intervention is to cut away the enlarged portions of the heart which complicate the cardiac problem, and thus to reduce the size of the heart. Replacement of part of the heart, especially the left ventricle, with an artificial ventricle to which the blood is diverted is yet another possibility.

Heart transplant remains the best solution to date. This intervention enjoys a high success rate (95% probability of survival for the first year, and 70% for the next eleven years). Unfortunately, there are extensive patient waiting lists.

The use of laser interventions is particularly helpful with older persons for whom traditional surgery may prove to be too great a risk.

REFERENCES

Aronow, W. & Tresch, D. (1997). Treatment of congestive heart failure in older persons. *JAGS, 45* (10), 1252-1257.

Bloom, B. (1990). Medical management and managing medical care: The dilemma of evaluating new technology. *American Heart Journal, 199* (3), 754-761.

DiGiovanna, A. G. (1994). *Human Aging.* New York: McGraw-Hill.

Oram, J.J. (1997). *Caring for the Fourth Age.* London: Armelle.

Perler, B. (1994). Vascular disease in the elderly patient. *Surgical Clinics of North America, 74* (1), 199-216.

Rowe, J.W., & Kahn, R. (1998). *Successful Aging.* New York: Pantheon.

Spence, A.D. (1995). *Biology of Human Aging.* Englewood Cliffs, NJ: Prentice-Hall.

Chapter 6

THE RESPIRATORY SYSTEM

The respiratory system functions within the context of several of the body systems. These include the skeletal, muscular, and circulatory systems. The circulatory and respiratory systems appear to operate as a unit. The primary function of the respiratory system to transport oxygen to the bloodstream and to remove carbon dioxide.

All cells within the body require a continuous supply of oxygen to carry out their various metabolic activities. The carbon dioxide that results from these activities must be removed. The organs of the respiratory system, in conjunction with those of the circulatory system, carry out these functions.

The delivery of oxygen throughout the body appears to be related to physical characteristics such as height. Very tall individuals, particularly men, seem to experience greater problems with regard to the respiratory system than do shorter men. The extended area which must be covered through respiration becomes increasingly problematic as the person grows older.

The organs of the respiratory system are affected more by environmental factors than are the organs of most other body systems. The principal organs of the respiratory system are the two lungs. Respiratory organs are constantly exposed to environmental factors, such as various pollutants in the air. The frequency of such onslaughts, along with respiratory infections, may well contribute to the premature aging of the human organism.

The respiratory system includes many protective devices to offset the intrusion of foreign particles. One of these is the cilia or hairs found principally in the nasal passages, with some in the throat and the mouth, which serve to keep out potentially harmful substances. Habits of breathing through the mouth can diminish the effectiveness of such protective measures.

The respiratory system includes the nasal cavity including the nasal passages and the olfactory system, the pharynx, the larynx, the trachea, the bronchi, the alveoli, and the lungs. As air is breathed in, it passes over moist areas and is heated before it passes into the lungs. The mucous membrane or lining of the pharynx and the throat, along with the cilia present, are all part of the protective barrier of the respiratory system. Substances caught in the cilia cause people to cough and sneeze to eject the particle.

The cilia when healthy resemble a field of wheat or grass in the spring when it stands erect and tall. Any form of pollution, such as smoking, or other destructive materials that enter the throat tend to bend the cilia downwards. Such continued onslaughts cause the cilia, much like grass, to remain bent and crushed. Such damage is permanent. The result of such bending is that the cilia no longer functions as a protective device, and substances once halted at the entrance of the throat, can now pass freely.

The malfunctioning cilia result in throat infections and respiratory diseases. The mucous membrane serves as a protective device, but bacteria like to live in warm, moist areas and generally inhabit these areas. Consequently, it is very difficult to overcome a disease once it centers itself in the lungs or anywhere in the respiratory tract. This is also the reason why many sexually transmitted diseases are difficult to treat and to overcome as they thrive in warm, dark, and moist areas. The throat presents a similar breeding ground. This is why infections of the throat often last for a long period of time as the irritation is more deep-seated.

An additional problem is presented by the fact that the ear, nose, mouth, and throat are all interlinked—they open into one another. Thus, diseases in one area spread easily to another, and because they are homogeneous areas—all dark and moist, they encourage the growth of bacteria which can move from one part to another almost endlessly. All of these passages interconnect,—so that an infection of the throat can easily move to the ear. It is for this reason that a person can experience hearing difficulties as the result of having had a cold. Otolaryngologists are physicians who specialize in problems of the ear, nose and throat.

The air from the nasal cavity moves down the pharynx, which has openings into the mouth, the ear, the esophagus or the trachea. Swallowing is an important function. People who have difficulty in swallowing are extremely uncomfortable. This disability may be due to malfunctioning of the muscles of the pharynx or possibly an obstruction due to cancer.

Swallowing and breathing are accomplished almost as single acts. Since persons are seldom conscious of either activity, they pass unnoticed. When a problem arises in this area, it can be quite disabling. Persons who cannot breathe or those for whom swallowing is difficult, this debility assumes enormous proportions. Since these are two actions which are performed simultaneously, it is difficult to disassociate them. Breathing and swallowing is accomplished at the same time. The purpose of such coordination is to eliminate the possibility that something could become stuck in the pharynx or might lodge somewhere in the respiratory system causing severe problems.

From the pharynx the air passes to the larynx, or the voice box. It then passes to the lungs and finally to the alveoli located at the base of each of the lungs. These alveoli are sac-like structures that hold reserve air which they empty periodically. This air, however, can become trapped in these sacs and become stale and prone to bacterial infection. Such infections can spread throughout the lungs and the entire respiratory system. The important exchange of air and the blood, which is a gaseous exchange, occurs in the alveoli. For this reason, it is important that the alveoli function properly.

The process of breathing relies upon the diaphragm which is located directly below the rib cage. The diaphragm in even very old people functions very well and is a tribute to the fact that those areas of the body that are constantly used remain, as a result, in optimal condition. In most instances, atrophy is the result of disuse.

For proper functioning, clean air is taken into the body, and stale air is released from the body. This process of taking in air is known as inspiration, and the letting out of stale air is expiration. In breathing in, the thoracic cavity is increased, and in breathing out, the thoracic cavity is diminished. The lungs, the diagram and muscles are involved in this process. An even exchange of air depends on healthy alveoli to ascertain that indeed such an exchange is taking place.

The rib cage which provides a protective covering to the lungs also is resilient and provides a certain "give" during inspiration and expiration. In older persons, such elasticity of the rib cage is lessened due to increased rigidity of the skeletal system, and the thoracic cavity does not expand and contract to the same degree. What is referred to as vital capacity is the amount of air that the person can take in during inspiration, and the amount of air the individual expels during expiration.

Alterations with Aging

Evidence of aging occurs when persons have difficulty in performing activities at the same rate or level at which they were able to perform when somewhat younger. People who are accustomed to running a number of miles per day, find that they can run fewer miles within the same time frame. Due to breathing problems, they are able to swim fewer laps. This does not indicate that persons as they grow older should eliminate certain activities, but rather that they perform them at less strenuous levels. According to the Italian geriatrician, Francesco Antonini, older persons should not be told not to climb mountains, but they should be exhorted to select smaller mountains. It is the level of the activity that should be the measure of what the person can accomplish.

Trachea and Bronchi

The cartilage in the walls of the trachea and bronchi become more rigid with aging. The smooth-muscle fibers in the walls of the bronchiole contain more fibrous connective tissue which cannot contract or to stretch as easily. Such changes, along with a reduced elasticity of the lungs and the wall of the thorax, decreases maximum breathing capacity and vital capacity. This alteration can begin as early as age 20. As vital capacity decreases, there is an increase in the volume of residual air in the lungs. An imbalance is created between the amount of fresh air and the amount of stale air exchanged.

Alveoli

There is a gradual breakdown of the walls between the alveoli. This tends to increase the size of the alveoli and to reduce the surface areas over which gaseous exchange takes place.

The alveoli are less elastic and do not expand and contract as easily. Air can become trapped in the alveoli, and this is particularly dangerous if the person smokes and lives or works in a heavily polluted environment. Much of the debris from such elements remains over protracted periods of time in the alveoli, and the oxygen passed through the blood contains elements of such contamination and is, thus, poor quality oxygen. Declining oxygen levels in the blood is the main age-related functional change in the respiratory system. Such internal pollution ultimately results in health problems.

Lungs

Lungs lose some of their elasticity with age. There is also an unequal distribution of air within the lungs. The volume of inspired air that reaches the region is insufficient to completely oxygenate the blood supply.

One such area where air and blood supply are not balanced is in the lower portions of the lungs. Due to reduced elasticity, the lungs of older persons often do not properly ventilate the alveoli. Thus, the oxygen-poor blood from the lungs can gradually dilute the blood from other regions, thereby reducing the level of oxygen saturation of arterial blood.

As a result, some regions of the body can be saturated appropriately, while others are not. In fact they may suffer from "oxygen poor" blood. This may account for the fatigue experienced by older persons. Insufficient amounts of oxygen in the blood that supplies the brain can lead to problems with mental functioning, such as memory loss. People who feel disoriented or dizzy, or persons who feel they cannot cope with the problems of everyday life are likely to be suffering from oxygen deprivation.

Structural Changes

The general structural changes which affect the body as people age, also alters the functioning of the respiratory system. Postural changes can affect the efficacy of the respiratory system. Erect posture has important psychological benefits, as well as improving respiratory functioning. People who develop habits of sitting in hunched positions or slumped in chairs or who do not stand erect develop rounding of the shoulders and a narrowing of the chest cavity. The posture of some older persons is so bent that they appear to be facing the ground, rather than facing forward. This accentuated downward posture gave rise to the saying that the grave is already beckoning the person. Such postural changes which cramp the lungs have a direct effect on the breathing capacity of the person.

Loss in height is common due to changes in the vertebrae, and persons who are in their 90s and 100s are much shorter than when they were younger. Stooping because of a dowager's hump makes women appear even shorter.

The rounding of the thoracic region of the vertebral column is due to the loss of calcium and a gradual weakening of muscles of the neck and back. These changes reduce the volume of the thoracic cavity, and it becomes difficult for the lungs to expand. Thus, breathing becomes more laborious for the older person. Since the cartilage that connects the ribs to the spinal column and sternum tends to calcify, joints become stiffer with age. These combined changes in the skeletal and respiratory systems make respiration more difficult and less efficient.

More muscular work is required to move air into and out of the lungs, and older persons tend to rely more on the diaphragm for inspiration. Older persons may find it more difficult to breathe when lying on their backs. This position increases intraabdominal pressure, which, coupled with the stiffness of the rib cage, makes it difficult to increase the volume of the thoracic cavity and to ventilate the lungs adequately. It is easier for older persons to breathe if they are elevated or supported by layers of pillows. It is also important to rotate persons who sleep on their sides or on their stomachs to prevent suffocation. Breathing is compromised by the presence of various disease states, along with senescence.

Caution has to be exercised in feeding persons who are bedfast due to the fact that breathing and swallowing are simultaneous actions. The breathing of persons in prone positions is already compromised, and the ingestion of food may create additional complications. Choking or the aspiration of food into the lungs can lead to serious consequences such as pneumonia or death.

Some bodily changes can be reversed or offset by a regular program of exercise. This is true of the skeletal, muscular, and circulatory systems. The respiratory system, however, is an exception. There are no muscles in the walls of the lungs. Only the diaphragm and the respiratory muscles of the chest wall could be strengthened by exercise.

Dysfunctions

Diseases of the respiratory system are common in old age and are frequently responsible for the limited respiratory reserve capacity and the development of dyspnea on exertion. It may also be aggravated by several changes in the respiratory system probably associated with the aging process. Older persons are also particularly vulnerable to developing respiratory tract infections.

Some of the dysfunctions of the respiratory system in older people may be due less to the aging process, but more to years of exposure to environmental factors, such as air pollution and smoking. Prolonged residence in industrialized cities can have baneful effects on the respiratory system.

Pulmonary disorders are divided into two categories: restrictive diseases or obstructive diseases. Restrictive diseases reduce the expansion of the lungs. In obstructive diseases the respiratory airways are compromised, and there is increased resistance to air flow.

Chronic Obstructive Pulmonary Disease

Chronic obstructive pulmonary disease (COPD) is a group of diseases in which there is a chronic obstruction in airflow to the lungs. Common symptoms are difficulty in breathing, coughing, and frequent expectoration. The symptoms become aggravated with advancing age. Men are more commonly affected.

COPD has been labeled as the most common chronic respiratory disorder. Once diagnosed, COPD is progressive and may lead to disability, usually due to dyspnea, at a relatively early age, approximately 60-80. The diagnosis is suspected in, but not limited to, persons with a history of several decades of cigarette smoking who present with non-specific respiratory symptoms.

Disorders blanketed by the term COPD include those conditions which are characterized by pulmonary insufficiency and limited airflow. In most individuals, both processes exist simultaneously. Such obstruction of the airways reduces the elimination of carbon dioxide and limits the amount of available oxygen in the body. The lack of available oxygen is manifested in COPD patients by hypoxia or abnormally low levels of oxygen in the blood.

The two most common chronic obstructive pulmonary diseases are chronic bronchitis and emphysema. Persons with these disorders tend to have a decrease in respiratory muscle efficiency paired with an increase in the actual work required in breathing. As the disease progresses, the ability to lead a normal life is diminished due to the extreme physical exhaustion which occurs during most forms of physical exertion. Later in the disease, even the smallest amount of exertion in everyday tasks can lead to exhaustion and shortness of breath. Nutrition intervention is need in severe COPD as resulting exhaustion may cause dyspnea and extreme fatigue making it difficult for the person to make and eat meals.

Malnutrition and COPD

Poor nutritional status contributes to and complicates pulmonary disease. Weight loss occurs, and it is difficult to isolate a single cause for weight loss because a number of factors are operative, including chronic mouth breathing, dyspnea, and depression. The inability to maintain adequate nutritional status increases the possibility of infection which is a common complication in pulmonary disease. Improving nutritional status is important when weaning patients from the respirator. Anorexia is another factor which promotes significant weight loss in most persons.

Treatment through Pulmonary Rehabilitation

Pulmonary rehabilitation is an important adjunct to standard medical therapy. Its primary goal is to restore persons to the highest possible functional state through a combination of exercise training, education, respiratory and chest physiotherapy techniques, and psychosocial support. Although pulmonary function generally does not change, exercise tolerance can improve, along with decreased symptoms of breathlessness, improved quality of life, and less requirement for health care services.

Preserving functional capacity and quality of life requires long-term commitments by the COPD patient. Smoking cessation, pulmonary rehabilitation, and medication are part of therapy required for COPD. Because COPD patients are commonly on numerous medications, it is important to note their effects on nutrition and appetite.

Environmental factors and age are primary causes of COPD. There are, however, some indications of possible genetic predisposition.

Cigarette smoking is considered to be a contributing factor in 80 percent of the cases. The person often assumes a stooped posture, even leaning on the elbows when in a sitting position. Breathing is labored and is often through pursed lips. The two most common chronic obstructive pulmonary diseases are emphysema and chronic bronchitis.

Emphysema

Emphysema is a disease in which there is actual destruction of some of the lungs. Excessive air accumulates in the lungs as they lose their ability to ventilate properly. The condition develops very gradually in response to other respiratory problems, such as chronic bronchitis, smoking, or other pulmonary irritants. There is some suggestion that persons can have a hereditary predisposition toward this disease. Emphysema is much more prevalent in older persons, and, although the disease may have been initiated in youth, it is only evidenced as the individual ages. As the disease progresses, it becomes irreversible, and results in death. Clinical diagnosis of emphysema in old age is more difficult than during youth.

Chronic irritation due to smoking, environmental pollution, or respiratory infections may eventually destroy the cilia of the mucous membrane lining the airways. The irritation leads to the production of large amounts of mucous within the airways. In an effort to rid the body of the heavy mucous secretions, the person develops a nagging cough. People who smoke excessively cough continuously upon first arising, and yet, such discomfort notwithstanding, their first act of the morning may be to smoke a cigarette.

Less air flows into and out of the alveoli during respiration, and the supply of fresh air is diminished. There is further the accumulation of debris from the pollution or cigarette smoking, and a resulting discoloration.

As a result of the trapped air, expiration requires muscular assistance, and persons deplete much of their total body energy when they exhale. An expanded "barrel chest" may be the end result. This is frequently observed in older men who are habitual smokers.

The level of oxygen in the blood may be too low to support mild physical activity. The elasticity of the lungs is diminished over time.

This results in a very low maximum breathing capacity and a high residual air volume. People suffering from emphysema are sometimes referred to as "pink puffers." The disease cannot be reversed and gradually worsens.

Emphysema overexerts the heart as it struggles to pump more blood to the lungs to compensate for the oxygen-poor blood leaving the lungs. Heart failure is a common cause of death.

Chronic Bronchitis

Chronic bronchitis is particularly common in old age. Chronic bronchitis is generally caused by bacterial infection or by irritants, such as smoke. Such persons often have a history of smoking. Chronic bronchitis is usually a result of long-term exposure to environmental irritants, the result of having lived or worked in polluted environments. In chronic bronchitis, as in emphysema, such irritation leads to excess mucous which can also produce a burning sensation. A lingering or unremitting cough may plague the individual. As the condition progresses, the mucous membrane may become swollen and partially obstruct the airways. Cyanosis often occurs in severe cases. Patients at this stage of the disease are sometimes referred to as "blue bloaters."

Pneumonia

The incidence of pneumonia is high among the older population, and its clinical presentation is usually atypical, making the diagnosis difficult. Pneumonia was once considered a disease that principally afflicted older persons. Before the advent of modern medical intervention, most older persons would die if they contracted pneumonia. Consequently, pneumonia was commonly referred to as the older person's best friend.

Pneumonia is an inflammation of the lower airways of the lung. Symptoms of pneumonia include fever, cough, and sputum production. Symptoms in older persons can also include confusion, loss of appetite, weakness, or a fall. Pneumonia is not limited to older persons, although it is a common disease of old age. Death due to pneumonia is more likely in persons over the age of 65.

Pneumonia is classified as community acquired or hospital acquired. Community-acquired pneumonia is usually caused by one of several viruses, especially the influenza viruses or the Pneumococcus bacterium. Hospital-acquired pneumonia is the more common type found in older persons. This may be due to their frequent confinement in hospitals or long-term care facilities.

The threat of aspiration pneumonia increases with age. This condition develops as the result of the inhalation of foods or other foreign bodies that obstruct a bronchus. The obstruction may cause a lung to collapse and fluids to accumulate, resulting in infection. Aspiration pneumonia is more common among bedfast persons, persons not fully conscious, or those having difficulty in swallowing.

Excessive alcohol consumption coupled with the ingestion of food can lead to aspiration pneumonia. The problem can occur when an individual vomits while lying on his or her back. Such accidental deaths can be prevented by ensuring that the person is placed on his or her side.

Persons who engage in life-threatening behavior or suicide often swallow objects to cause obstructions. To accomplish this end, people have swallowed large pieces of food, facial tissue, toilet tissue, and dollar bills.

Tuberculosis

Tuberculosis was once a more common disease. Throughout the world, hospitals and sanitariums to treat persons suffering from this disease were commonplace. Sanitaria were usually located in elevated or mountainous regions. Rest and relaxation, along with breathing purer air, was the prescribed treatment. Many patients had a history of leaving and returning to sanitaria, and eventually dying of the disease. Entire families might be infected by this disease. Those who did not go to sanitoria but remained at home, spent years in bed as invalids. Persons who could engage in partial activities soon became fatigued, and altered their lives between limited activity and periods of bedrest. As medical knowledge grew in the detection and treatment of tuberculosis (especially the development of antibiotics), and standards of living and working improved, this disease came under control. There appears, however, to be a current upsurge of this disease. This may, in part, be due to the increase in the incidence of AIDS.

Those who do develop symptoms can usually be treated with various drug therapies. Tuberculosis of the lungs is the most common form of this disease. Early symptoms are not always obvious to the individual. Symptoms include weight loss, cough, difficulty breathing, weakness, a pink flush in the cheeks and fever. A positive diagnosis requires a skin test, chest x-ray films, and sputum cultures.

Even before the advent of the AIDS epidemic, tuberculosis was a significant health problem for older persons. The likelihood of their having inhaled the bacterium in their youth is very high. The bacteria may have remained dormant over the years without manifesting signs of the disease. As the person ages, and there is a reduction in the effectiveness of the immune system, the lung can become reinfected. This reactivation tuberculosis is generally what occurs in older persons.

The reactivation of disease in old age is true not only of tuberculosis, but it is the case with several other diseases as well. Chickenpox can be reactivated as herpes or shingles in older persons. Women who become diabetic during pregnancy may experience a reactivation of diabetes when they grow old. There may well be additional varieties of bacteria and viruses that can remain dormant for long periods of time.

Pulmonary Embolism

An embolus is a blood clot or other substance that breaks free and begins to travel within the blood vessels. The major danger of an embolus is that, at some point, it may lodge in a narrow area and partially or completely block the vessel. This diminishes or cuts off the blood flow, and the tissues may deteriorate or die.

A pulmonary embolism is a clot that blocks a section of a pulmonary artery. Symptoms of pulmonary embolism include shortness of breath, rapid heart rate, anxiety, chest pain, and expectoration of blood.

Emboli are more common in older persons who lead sedentary lives or who are bedfast. Bedfast patients have a higher probability of developing blood clots because the rate of blood flow is reduced. Anticoagulant drugs are usually prescribed for the condition.

Such age related changes contribute to a reduction in the amount of oxygen reaching the lung capillaries in older persons, thereby reducing older persons' capacity for physical activity. Older persons may experience fatigue more easily and have to restrict the extent of their participation in vocational or recreational activities due to oxygen deprivation. Such deprivation can exert consequences as serious as those experienced by food deprivation.

The health problems associated with the respiratory system are unusually not in and of themselves life-threatening. It is when they are associated with life-style behaviors, such as smoking, that are harmful to the system, that real dangers emerge.

Environmental Factors

Older persons who have spent the major part of their lives in large cities find that as they grow older there is increasing damage to their respiratory system due to air pollution. Persons living in large cities are encouraged to wear face masks; preventive measures are becoming commonplace in congested areas of large cities such as Milan and Tokyo. Pollution of the atmosphere is directly related to shortened life expectancy. On the other hand, persons who live in rural areas have longer life expectancies. It is unclear how many deaths of older persons who reside in inner cities may be linked to environmental pollution.

Technology and Interventions

Recent advances in video technology and endoscopic instrumentation have expanded the use of thoracoscopy from diagnosis to treatment of pulmonary disease. Because of advances in endoscopic surgical equipment and anesthetic technology, surgical treatment via thoracoscopy is now possible. Thoracoscopy was introduced more than 80 years ago for the diagnosis of pleural disease. This technique was limited until recent advances allowed thoracic surgeons to have greater visualization and mobility within the chest.

Lung Cancer

Lung cancer is the leading cause of cancer deaths in the United States. Lung cancer risk increases with the intensity and duration of cigarette smoking, the depth of inhalation, and the tar and nicotine content of the cigarettes. The overall survival rates for patients with all stages of lung cancer are low. Patients with lung cancer may not receive surgical treatment if their preoperative pulmonary function tests reveal chronic obstructive pulmonary disease (COPD). Nearly 90 percent of patients with lung cancer also have COPD, and 20 percent of these patients have severe pulmonary dysfunction.

With the introduction of lung volume reduction surgery (LVRS) in 1993, the patient selection criteria for lung surgery are being reassessed. Patients with emphysema are benefitting from surgical resection of their hyperinflated lung tissue, and many patients with lung cancer and COPD now are undergoing combined LVRS and pulmonary nodule resection. The postoperative improvements in these patients' pulmonary function partially outweigh the surgical risks of the combined procedures. Previously some patients with emphysema and who also had lung nodules were denied surgery because of the severity of their pulmonary dysfunction.

REFERENCES

Adams, F. V. (1998). *The Breathing Disorders Source Book.* Los Angeles: Lowell House.

Allen, G., & DeRose, J. (1997). Pulmonary nodule resection during lung volume reduction surgery. *AORN Journal, 66*(5), 808-818.

Aspen Reference Group. (1998). *Dieticians' patient education manual.* Gaithersburg, MD: Aspen Reference Group.

Celli, B. R. (1998). Pathophysiology of chronic obstructive pulmonary disease. *Respiratory Care Clinics of North America, 2*(3), 359-370.

Chapman, K., & Winter, L. (1996).COPD: Using nutrition to prevent respiratory function decline. *Geriatrics, 51*(12), 37-42.

Colt, H., Ries, A., et al. (1997). Analysis of chronic obstructive pulmonary disease referrals for lung volume reduction surgery. *Journal of Cardiopulmonary Rehabilitation, 17,* 248-252.

Dantzker, D. R. (1989). Fresh ideas on COPD. *Medical World News, 30*(20), 53.

Kart, S. K., Metress, E. K., & Metress, S. P. (1992). *Human Aging and Chronic Disease.* Boston: Jones & Bartlett.

Miller, L. D., Allen, S. M., et al. (1992). Videothoracoscopic wedge excision of the lung. *The Society of Thoracic Surgeons, 79* (9), 572-578.

Oram, J. J. (1997). *Caring for the Fourth Age.* London: Armelle.

Phillips, Y. Y., & Hnatiuk, O. W. Diagnosing and monitoring the clinical course of chronic obstructive pulmonary disease. *Respiratory Care Clinics of North America, 4*(3), 371-389.

Postma, D. S. (1998). When can an exacerbation of COPD be treated at home? *The Lancet, 351* (9119), 1827-1828.

Resnikoff, P. M., & Ries, A. L. Maximizing functional capacity. Pulmonary rehabilitation and adjunctive measures. *Respiratory Care Clinics of North America,4*(3), 475-492.

Spence, A. D. (1995). *Biology of Human Aging* (2nd ed.). Englewood Cliffs, NJ: Prentice-Hall.

Utell, M., & Samet, J. (1990). Environmentally mediated disorders of the respiratory tract. *Medical Clinics of North America, 74* (2), 291-306.

Chapter 7

THE DIGESTIVE SYSTEM

People are living longer, and an increasing body of evidence is demonstrating that preventive measures begun early in life and maintained throughout life can significantly reduce the prevalence of acute and chronic diseases in old age. These measures include diet modification, regular exercise, smoking avoidance, and periodic medical screening, especially for blood pressure and cancer. At the same time, because of increases in life expectancy during the last 50 years, a generation of persons is growing up with the knowledge that if they practice healthy life behaviors, they are likely to live to reach advanced ages. Efforts to extend knowledge of behaviors that promote health and prevent crippling and chronic disease at older ages are thus becoming more important. Behavior alone cannot ensure longevity; however, the social and economic context is extremely important. People who cannot afford nourishing food, adequate housing, and essential medical care cannot live healthy life-styles even if they know how to do so.

Much like other systems within the body, the digestive system relies upon other bodily systems to function appropriately. The digestive system generally presents few major problems to older persons. The threat of cancer of the digestive system, however, increases with age. Frequent complaints, nonetheless, center about gastrointestinal disorders such as indigestion, heartburn, loss of appetite, and constipation. Some of these disorders can be linked to items in the diet such as spices (tomatoes are acidic), eating late in the evening or at night, the amount of liquid ingested, and the use of alcohol. Unfortunately, many of these digestive disturbances occur at night and interfere with the person's sleep.

The digestive system consists of a long tube known as the gastrointestinal tract. The main function of the digestive system is to change the composition of food to a form that can be assimilated by the body cells.

The digestive process begins in the mouth, with the food being chewed by the teeth, maneuvered about the mouth by the tongue, and being acted upon by enzymes located in the mouth which initiates the breakdown of food. The saliva is important in this preparation of the food to move from the mouth, to the pharynx, to the esophagus, down to the stomach, the small and large intestines, and finally to the anus for waste removal.

As people age, there is a reduction in the secretions of the digestive glands. The muscles in the walls of the tract become weaker, and there is a reduction in the strength of its contractions. Other changes in the digestive system reflect the normal aging changes of the entire organism.

Mouth

A common problem for older persons is oral health care. Many persons lose their teeth by the age of 65, or they wear or require dentures. While oral health care has improved, and older persons are more conscious of its importance, major concern still exists with regard to periodontal or gum disease.

Periodontal disease is an inflammation which can destroy the periodontal membrane that lines the tooth socket. Consequently, the tooth becomes loose, and the gum draws away from the tooth. This forms a pocket on the gums in which bacteria and food particles collect and eventually cause an infection. Periodontal disease may be, in part, a form of nutritional osteoporosis due to a deficiency in calcium.

The absence of teeth or the wearing of uncomfortable dentures compromises the older person's ability to chew. Difficult or painful mastication can cause people to select softer and more easily chewable foods to the detriment of nutritional balance. The health of the digestive system may also be affected as it requires the presence of some fiber content in food. Softer foods can lack fiber or bulk and can cause chronic constipation.

There is a reduction in the amount of saliva present in the oral cavity. Older persons' mouths feel drier. Dryness of the mouth can be linked to a systemic dysfunction or to the use of medications. The sensation of taste can be altered when sufficient amounts of saliva are no longer present. The role of saliva in oral health care is to cleanse the mouth and teeth. Reduced saliva affects these functions as well.

Mouth breathing also dries the mouth. Difficulty in masticating foods in the absence of sufficient saliva can alter food habits and may lead to malnutrition and constipation. Dry mouth is such a common problem that saliva substitutes such as mouth sprays have been developed.

The tongue plays an important role in preparing the food to descend into the pharynx. The tongue moves food about the mouth, and squashes the food down into small portions for the teeth to break down. The tongue reaches all recesses of the mouth interior and piles the food against the teeth. This mashing of food is an important preparation of the food for the initiation of the digestive process.

Older persons frequently complain that food is not as flavorful as it once was. Decreased amounts of saliva are responsible for some loss of taste. As part of the normal aging process, there is in addition an atrophy of taste buds. There are approximately 70 percent fewer taste buds present at age 70 than there were at age 30. A diminished sense of taste can affect a person's eating behavior. Loss of appetite or general disinterest in food can eventually affect nutritional status and overall physical and mental health.

Life-style factors such as cigarette smoking and extensive use of alcohol can also alter the sense of taste. Persons with lifetime habits of cigarette smoking admit to having difficulty in distinguishing various foods.

Diminishment in the functioning of the sense of smell can also affect appetite levels. The aroma of food in preparation is often a stimulant for eating. In this manner, the sense of taste and smell play a complementary role as both are chemical senses. The protective qualities of the sense of smell also serve to dissuade persons from eating contaminated or ill-smelling food items and thus avoiding potential hazards of food poisoning. In older persons the sense of smell does not appear to function as efficiently. Such losses, however, are gradual in nature.

Esophagus

Older persons can experience problems in swallowing and esophageal pain. Neurological disorders can bring on swallowing problems. The movement of food from the esophagus into the stomach is controlled by the esophageal sphincter at the entrance into the stomach. The sphincter can weaken with age. In such instances, food moves back up into the esophagus. This condition is known as heartburn. Gas from the stomach can also pass through the weakened sphincter back up the esophagus causing frequent and sometimes painful belching.

Stomach

The mucous membrane lining the stomach tends to thin with age, and contractions of the stomach are diminished. The rate of emptying solids from the stomach does not alter with age, but liquids may remain in the stomach longer than in younger persons.

Small and Large Intestines

The walls of both the large and small intestine become weaker as people age. A condition known as diverticulosis can occur in the wall of the large intestine. This results from the formation of outpockets in the weakened large intestinal wall which can lead to infections.

The amount of bacterial flora alters in the large intestine as people grow older. Such bacterial growth is beneficial to the proper functioning of the digestive system. Any changes in bacterial growth may lead to nutritional deficiencies.

Pancreas

As people age, there may be an increase in the incidence of obstruction of the pancreatic ducts which prevents the passage of pancreatic juice to the small intestine. Such secretions can become lodged within the pancreas, and can cause inflammation of the pancreas or pancreatitis. This condition can lead to chronic disturbances of the digestive system and become quite debilitating.

Liver

Lipofuscin is commonly found in the liver cells of older persons. The structural changes of the liver with aging probably do not greatly affect its functioning as new liver cells regenerate very quickly, and the liver has a large measure of redundancy. Even when as much as 80 percent of the organ is removed, the remainder can still adequately provide for the needs of the body.

The ability of the liver to metabolize certain drugs alters as people advance in age. The reactions of older persons to certain drugs may vary considerably from the reactions of much younger individuals. Drug dosage levels should be administered in accordance with the person's age. Drugs prescribed for older persons should be routinely reevaluated. This is also true of drugs which a person may have taken over a long period of time for a chronic condition.

Cirrhosis of the liver is the fifth most common cause of death in the United States. It is closely associated with chronic alcoholism which is an important disorder in the elderly.

Dysfunctions

Although the digestive system operates without major problems well into old age, some common non-life threatening conditions increase. These include loss of appetite, dry mouth, belching, heartburn, difficulty in swallowing, and decreased acidity of digestive juices.

Hiatal Hernia

The esophagus enters the abdominal cavity through an opening in the diaphragm called a hiatus. A hiatal hernia occurs when the upper portion of the stomach protrudes from the abdominal cavity into the thoracic cavity through the hiatus. The condition is more common in females and in obese individuals over the age of 50. Older women are more often affected than are men.

Although available treatments do not correct the problem, symptoms can be significantly reduced. The condition is generally treated with medications. The consumption of smaller more broadly spaced meals is recommended. Elevation of the head and chest during sleep appears to relieve symptoms. Programs of weight reduction are also beneficial.

Cancer

One of the more serious problems of the digestive system is the rise in the numbers of malignant cancers (carcinomas) of the digestive system with age. Cancer of the esophagus is most common among men who smoke.

Stomach cancer is also more common in men over the age of 60. Some symptoms of stomach cancer include loss of appetite, weight loss, and a general feeling of malaise. Since the symptoms are non-specific, the diagnosis of cancer of the digestive tract is difficult and problematic. Persons may not consult a physician until the disease has substantially progressed. Furthermore, people resort to self-medication for extended periods of time which can be more damaging than beneficial. Medical advice is often sought after the disease progresses to a more advanced stage and symptoms become more severe. Symptoms of stomach cancer can include nausea, severe abdominal pain, and blood in the feces.

Some forms of malignant cancers of the pancreas, liver, and gallbladder also increase with age. Cancer does not often develop in the small intestine. Cancer of the large intestine and rectum is common in men and women and is often fatal. It occurs most frequently after the age of 70.

The high death rate from cancer of the large intestine can also be attributed to the fact that it is usually diagnosed only after it has reached an advanced stage of development. Early intervention is possible since a high percentage of cancers in the large intestine can be detected during a proctoscopic examination. If the tumors are removed surgically during their early stages, the likelihood of survival improves dramatically.

Diverticulitis

Diverticula are tiny pouches that develop in the wall of the intestines that protrude outward through the muscular layer. Fecal matter can collect in these pouches, and the region can become inflamed or infected. This condition is then referred to as diverticulitis. The incidence of diverticulitis increases gradually with age. It is more prevalent in women.

The symptoms can include abdominal pain accompanied by diarrhea or constipation, and blood in the feces. Diverticulitis is usually managed with a special high-fiber diet and antibiotic medications.

This disease is found more frequently in developed countries. Diets low in fiber are generally considered to be the cause. Diets high in fiber tend to move more quickly through the intestinal tract, and food remains in the tract for only several days. Those groups who consume diets low in fiber can have food lodged in the intestinal tract for as long as a week. Such a condition can also lead to the development of hemorrhoids.

Constipation

The infrequent or difficult evacuation of feces from the bowel is a condition known as constipation. The hard feces that develop are the result of the slow movement of digestive waste products through the large intestine. As these materials continue to linger in the colon, they absorb more water and become even drier and harder. This condition can be avoided by consuming a high-fiber diet, drinking sufficient quantities of water, and exercising. Constipation is a common complaint among older women. One major cause of constipation in older persons is a heavy reliance on laxative use.

It is important that persons do not constantly upset their normal defecation cycle. Persons who maintained regular bowel habits throughout life are unlikely to experience constipation in old age.

Fecal Incontinence

Fecal incontinence is not as common as urinary incontinence. It has, however, severe traumatic psychological effects on the person and drastically curtails social contacts. The diminished capability to regulate one's bowel movements is a problem for many older persons, particularly residents in long-term care facilities.

Health problems related to incontinence can be obviated through proper procedures of hygiene. It can, however, be very damaging to an individual's self-esteem. No one's self image includes being incontinent. Fecal incontinence is an impairment of the ability to control the external anal sphincter and the striated muscles forming the pelvic floor. Such loss of control can result from diseases such as cancer or neurological problems.

Some persons experience fecal incontinence during phases of an illness. Not infrequently, fecal incontinence is drug induced. It has been said that people are born incontinent and die incontinent.

Hemorrhoids

Many older persons suffer from hemorrhoids which are swollen or ruptured blood vessels of the lower bowel. They may be present within the anal canal or around the anus. Hemorrhoids can cause pain, itching, or bleeding. They are usually caused by constipation.

In general, eight to ten glasses of water a day and a diet that is balanced but bulk-producing can reduce or prevent hemorrhoids. The increased incidence of hemorrhoids in industrial societies has been linked to low-fiber diets.

Nutrition

Water Balance

An important aspect of overall nutrition is water balance. Several factors conspire to put older people at a relatively high risk of dehydration. For example, older people have a lower capacity to conserve water through the kidneys, as well as a significantly lower sensation of thirst. This is particularly problematic in acute illnesses accompanied with fever, such as common colds and flu, which increase the risk of dehydration even further. Dehydration can also increase the risk of flu-related complications (such as sinusitis and pneumonia).

Older persons should consume about one and a half to two quarts of fluid per day. This need not be consumed as water alone, but can include juices and other beverages that consist mainly of water.

Recommended Dietary Allowances and Dietary Reference Intakes

Food and eating behavior are part of an individual's sociocultural background. Food serves many cultural and socially significant functions. The quantity, quality, and combination of foods eaten reflect the life-style of the older person.

Relatively little is known about the effects of age on requirements for specific nutrients. Recommended dietary allowances (RDAs), promulgated by the Food and Nutrition Board of the U.S. National Academy of Sciences since 1941, define the level of essential nutrients adequate to meet the known nutrient needs of practically all healthy persons. RDAs were designed to avoid nutrient deficiency and associated diseases. RDAs are provided for protein, eleven vitamins, and seven mineral and energy requirements. Currently the RDAs are being replaced by Dietary Reference Intakes (DRIs), a term that encompasses the former RDAs as well as issues such as tolerable upper intake levels. Also, in a major advance, DRIs are being developed for various age groups, including separate recommendations for ages 51 through 70 and over 70.

Fat

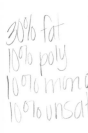

Older persons should follow the same guidelines for fat intake as younger people are given: that is, no more than 30 percent of total daily calories from fat, with no more than 10 percent from saturated fat, 10 percent from polyunsaturated fat, and 10 percent from monounsaturated fat. Since cholesterol does not seem to carry as much risk for the elderly as in younger adults, limitation of cholesterol intake does not seem necessary in most older persons.

Carbohydrates

Dietary carbohydrates, sugars and starches, often found in "white" foods, i.e., sugar, potatoes, pasta, and bread, should supply 55 to 60 percent of daily calories. Unfortunately, most people get no more than 45 to 50 percent in their diets. The emphasis should be on complex carbohydrates, which contain soluble fiber and are found in some fruits, peas, beans, and lentils. These can help reduce the incidence of constipation and formation of another gastrointestinal problem known as colonic diverticula. Dietary fiber also reduces blood fat and sugar levels and may be important in preventing heart disease.

Protein   12% protein

Older people may need more protein than younger people. Protein is found in meats, fish, poultry, eggs, and dairy products. Approximately 12 percent of total calories should come from protein. While the average American diet contains more than this amount, many elderly do not eat enough protein because of their inability to chew or to afford meats; other compromising factors include the inability or lack of desire to cook. Infections, surgery, and metabolic stresses, all relatively common in older people, also increase protein requirements. Chronic dietary protein insufficiency may reduce the ability to fight disease and to heal wounds, and may reduce the older individual's overall muscle strength.

Vitamins

Vitamin B6

Many older people are deficient in vitamin B6, which can impair the ability to fight disease, and can lead to increase in homocysteine, a risk factor for heart disease and stroke. Good dietary sources of B6 are chicken, fish, kidney, liver, pork, eggs, and to a lesser extent unmilled rice, soybeans, oats, whole wheat products, peanuts, and walnuts.

Folic Acid and Vitamin B12

Folic acid and B12 intake in older adults is a topic of great interest. One of the most common changes that affect nutrition in old age occurs in the gastrointestinal tract. Atrophic gastritis, a wearing out of the lining of the stomach leading to lower levels of acid secretion, is seen in approximately 35 percent of men and women by age 80. This problem leads to decreased absorption of folic acid and vitamin B12. Other factors, such as poverty and use of many medications, are also associated with poor folic acid intake in older people.

Folic acid (or folate) is found in a wide variety of foods such as leafy vegetables, liver, yeast, and some fruits. A number of older persons have low blood levels of this important nutrient. Low or even low-normal folic acid levels are associated with high levels of the amino acid homocysteine, which is a risk factor for heart disease and stroke, and possibly dementia.

Vitamin B12 deficiency among older persons is also common and is associated with anemia, neurologic disorders, and other major health problems. Low intake of red and organ meats, major dietary sources of vitamin B12, is an important risk factor for vitamin B12 deficiency among less affluent older adults.

Fat-Soluble Vitamins

In general, the older population should be at lower risk of deficiency in fat-soluble vitamins such as A, D, K, and E, because of their ability to store these vitamins in the liver and fat tissue. Since vitamin D derives from foods and from sunlight exposure, homebound or institutionalized older persons have limited dietary intake and often lack adequate sunlight exposure. Good dietary sources of vitamin D include fortified milk, butter, eggs, and seafood. Vitamin D is also important in increasing the absorption of calcium from foods.

Oral Health

Oral health is an essential factor in maintaining the general health and well-being of the elderly. Poor oral health is a major contributor to malnutrition, loss of strength, poor general health, and facial disfigurement. Furthermore, when oral health declines, embarrassment and social withdrawal often follow. Without social relationships, a downward spiral of self-esteem and general health is likely.

Older individuals whose oral cavities have been damaged by dental disease can benefit from recent advances in dental technology by which teeth may be restored or replaced by prostheses and by which the periodontal tissues (bone and gingiva or gums) may be restored to health.

It has long been established that diet and nutrition are important factors in both the cause and prevention of oral disease. Loss of teeth may be a higher predictor of inadequate nutrition than are demographic factors such as living alone. As teeth are lost, the nutritional quality of the diet declines.

Although the older population utilizes the greatest proportion of health care dollars, it has the lowest utilization rate of dental services at the time of life when the need for dental treatment is the greatest. Clinical examinations of older persons have shown a discrepancy between actual dental need and dental need as perceived by elders themselves. Many older persons believe that they must accept dental pain and tooth loss as part of the aging process. One might expect that the 5 percent of older persons who reside in nursing homes where their medical needs are met would have a higher rate of utilization of dental services than older persons living in the community. Unfortunately, this is not the case.

Technology, Prevention, and Intervention

It is now clear that dental caries (decay) in adults can be reduced through proper nutrition, removal of dental plaque through brushing and flossing, and use of fluoride. Dental implants have now been used successfully in some cases.

Despite the recent advances in dental technology, utilization of dental services by elders remains low in comparison with that of other age groups. No one is too old for dental treatment. A healthy 90 year old can have dental implants as successfully as a 50 year old, even where there is little or no alveolar bone (bone which supports the teeth or denture) remaining.

When proper medical precautions are taken, comprehensive dental care is as possible for an older patient, as it is for a younger patient. With appropriate treatment such as root canal therapy, implants, crowns and bridges, and periodontal treatment, older persons can keep their teeth for a lifetime.

If teeth are lost, a dental prosthesis such as a complete or partial denture can be provided. Although a prosthesis is never as good as one's own teeth, an individual can learn to use it effectively and continue to function well.

Older persons need to be educated to the importance of dental care for overall health. Health care professionals have the obligation to inform older persons of the new procedures and materials currently available to restore oral health and to maximize optimal functioning.

Dental Devices for the Elderly

Prosthetic replacements for dental structures date back to the earliest period of recorded history. The prosthetic devices were initially designed to compensate for lost chewing efficiency and to better one's appearance; however, advances in technology and therapeutics, reflecting the general advances in science, commerce, and the arts, resulted in dental prostheses being designed and fabricated to be more compatible with mouth tissue and more conducive to speech, deglutition, and respiration. The cosmetic aspects of dental prostheses were known to the early Egyptians, Greeks, and Romans, especially in the context of rituals of death, mummification, and funereal face masks. Edentulous mouths were plumped with artifacts to improve the face's appearance. Wrought gold, ivory, animal bone, and wood were hand-carved by artisans to replace a lost tooth or even a complete set of teeth.

There is also ample evidence of frequent attempts to transplant teeth from humans and even animals as early as the seventeenth century. Because these attempts at transplanting teeth were costly, they were considered only by the wealthy. With the development of vulcanization in the early nineteenth century and the firing of porcelain for teeth late in that century, artificial devices for replacing teeth become popular and affordable for middle-class and working-class people.

Nonetheless, the popularity of dental prostheses increased only very slowly because of the popular myth that losing teeth was a natural adjunct to growing old. It was not considered unattractive or unhealthy for a person to be partially or completely edentulous. Time, however, has changed these attitudes. New knowledge in biomedical science, technology, and therapeutics has increased the mean expectation of longevity from 50 years or more in the late nineteenth century to 80 years or more today. Although more accessible dental care, increases in economic status, and public entitlement for dental care have reduced the percentage of lost teeth per person, the increases in population and in life expectancy have left a large need for dental prostheses. Currently, there are approximately 35 million people who are edentulous in one form or another; another 15 million who have lost more than 75 percent of their teeth will become completely edentulous within the next decade.

The major impetus for providing dental care and dental prostheses is pragmatic. It is assumed that dental prostheses will make the wearer look more attractive, speak more effectively, and select and ingest more nutritious foods, as well as enhance his or her educational, vocational, and social options. Dental prostheses are essential to good physical and mental health.

The dental prosthesis also provides better control and modification of the airflow for speech and respiratory function. Prolonged chewing made possible by the prosthesis may improve secretion, taste, and smell differentiation. In addition, the aesthetic improvement is associated with a significant improvement in self-esteem and more active social participation. A dental prosthesis is successful when it facilitates normal speaking, chewing, and swallowing; does no harm to the residual tissues; is serviceable, can be altered or adjusted to compensate for changing biologic processes; and, maintains tissues in good health with minimum additional costs.

REFERENCES

Butler, R. N., & Brody, J. A., (Eds.). (1995). *Delaying the Onset of Late-Life Dysfunction.* New York: Springer.

Cain, W., & Stevens, J. (1990). Missing ingredients: Aging and the discrimination of flavor. *Journal of Nutrition for the Elderly, 9,* 3-15.

DiGiovanna, A. G. (1994). *Human Aging.* New York: McGraw-Hill.

Hamdy, R. C. (1984). *Geriatric Medicine.* Philadelphia: Bailliere Tindall.

Harris, R. (Ed.). (1983). *Medical devices and instrumentation for the elderly.* Arlington, VA: Association for the Advancement of Medical Instrumentation.

Kart, C. S. (1997). *The Realities of Aging.* Boston: Allyn & Bacon.

Lesnoff-Caravaglia, G. (Ed.). (1988). *Aging in a Technological Society.* New York: Human Sciences Press.

Lesnoff-Caravaglia, G. (Ed.). (1987). *Handbook of Applied Gerontology.* New York: Human Sciences Press.

Rowe, J.W., & Kahn, R. (1998). *Successful Aging.* New York: Pantheon.

Spence, A. D. (1995). *Biology of Human Aging.* Englewood Cliffs, NJ: Prentice-Hall.

Walter, J., & Soliah, L. (1995). Sweetener preference among non-institutionalized older adults. *Journal of Nutrition for the Elderly, 14,* 1-13.

Chapter 8

THE URINARY SYSTEM

Human beings are born incontinent and must learn to be continent. The urinary system is seldom consciously considered, and is, by and large, taken for granted until a problem surfaces. The functions associated with urination are performed perfunctorily and without much thought given to their execution. Urinary disorders, however, are significant causes of death and morbidity in the elderly.

The urinary system is considerably altered as aging proceeds. Many of its changes are primarily related to changes in the tissues of the urinary system. However, it is closely related to other systems, especially the circulatory and endocrine systems, and responds to changes in them as well.

The primary function of the urinary system is generally considered to be the excretion of urine. Urine serves as an extremely important means of removing from the body a variety of waste products and other potentially toxic substances. When there is the signal to urinate, it is important that this function be performed as soon as possible in order to rid the body of such wastes. Their prolonged stay in the body can result in deleterious effects and become potential health hazards. Delay in urination, especially as is the practice with many women or forced upon school children, can only compromise individual health.

Several body systems are involved in helping to remove waste products or unneeded substances from the body. Through the digestive system cells receive the nutrients they need to function properly and to eliminate waste products following digestion. The respiratory system supplies oxygen to the body for cellular metabolism and eliminates carbon dioxide, a waste product of cellular metabolism. The principal excretory organs of the urinary system are the kidneys. They play a critical role in maintaining the homeostasis of the body. This is done through the regulation of water content within the body and sustaining the balance of additional substances which may either need to be retained in the body or excreted.

Kidney dysfunction is an important, but not universal, aspect of aging. However, the aged kidney's limited ability to compensate for homeostatic challenges presented by other diseases is probably of greater significance. The changes that take place in the aging kidney do not appear to be handicapping in themselves. When disease of the kidney or other tissue challenges the elderly, the lowered reserve of renal function can have serious effects. The kidney's homeostatic role is clearly vital. Even relatively common events, such as diarrhea and vomiting, can be life-threatening to older persons.

As people age, renal function declines as does the ability to filter. Plasma flow, tubular absorption and excretion are also functions of the kidney that are affected. As the person ages, the kidneys actually become smaller.

When one kidney is removed, it is characteristic for the other one to show compensatory hypertrophy (grow larger) with an important increase in functional capacity. The older an individual is, the less compensatory hypertrophy occurs; moreover, the retained kidney already has the reduced functioning concomitant with age. These facts are relevant when considering the age of kidney donors for transplantation, since older individuals are more threatened by the loss of a kidney.

The urinary bladder, ureters, and urethra are structures that depend on the proper function of their muscular elements. Loss of muscle tone results in difficulty in emptying the bladder, or, in other cases, incontinence, the involuntary loss of urine. The bladder capacity for urine volume also diminishes with age.

Urinary incontinence is common among the elderly, especially in women over the age of 65. Cultural stigma and embarrassment have prevented many people from acknowledging and reporting the problem, although it is usually treatable. It is about half as frequent among men, but men suffer much more from an opposite problem, involuntary continence. In older males, the prostate gland surrounding the urethra commonly enlarges to constrict the urethra. The prostate gland is also part of the reproductive system.

Urinary tract infections are also quite common in the older population. Urinary tract infections and pneumonia were found to be responsible for more than half of all infections in health care settings. The most commonly associated causes of urinary tract infections include a lack of handwashing between patient contacts by health care professionals, close proximity to others with catheters, poor positioning of drainage bags, and poor catheter insertion techniques. Urinary tract infections are much more prevalent among women than men and is attributable to such facts as the tendency toward having a short urethra in close proximity to the rectal opening, the absence of prostatic fluid and its bacteriostatic qualities, and urethral compression by an enlarging uterus in pregnancy. Several other factors influence the rate of urinary tract infection including socioeconomic status, personal hygiene practices, and analgesic abuse.

Urinary tract infections are usually treated with an antibiotic or antimicrobial treatment therapy in order to insure that the infection will not spread to other areas. In addition to the drug therapy, increases in fluid intake is recommended to dilute the urine, to increase urine flow, and to prevent dehydration. To prevent urinary tract infections, older persons should be encouraged to stay active and to wear loose fitting undergarments and clothing. Prevention is difficult due to the fact that many occurrences are due directly to bacteria.

Kidneys

One alteration in the kidneys which has serious consequences for older persons is the reduced capability of the kidneys to concentrate urine. An additional change, equally significant, is the diminished ability to resorb glucose and sodium. There is also a decrease in blood supply to the kidneys.

Impaired tubular functioning in the kidneys may affect the elimination of substances such as drugs. Changes in the kidneys that are caused by the process of aging have a direct effect on the amount and frequency of drug administration in the older population. As life expectancy continues to be extended, it is important that drugs prescribed for older persons be adjusted periodically so that there is a close match between the aged organism and drug dosage levels. Many drugs are inappropriate for use with older persons, and the dosages of drugs may have been established on younger age groups.

Despite such possible changes, the kidneys are generally not seriously impaired as people grow old.

Bladder and Urethra

As a general change of the muscular system, the muscles in the walls of the bladder and urethra become weakened and are less elastic. Such muscle weakness, along with age-related changes in connective tissue, cause changes in the bladder. The expansion and contraction of the bladder is reduced.

The bladder of an older person has a capacity of less than half that of a young adult. As a result of muscular weakness, the bladder of the older person may retain as much as half as residual urine—urine retained in the bladder after urination. A problem older persons face is that the desire to urinate is not noticed until the bladder is practically full. In younger people the micturition reflex or desire to urinate is activated when the bladder is half full, but in the elderly this does not occur until the bladder is near capacity. The defect in this reflex may be due to age changes in the cerebral cortex or to the damage associated with a tumor. Frequent urination and extreme urgency to urinate in older persons are results of decreases in bladder size and a delayed micturition reflex. Pressure on the urethra due to obesity increases the need to urinate more frequently. These conditions are annoying to the person even if they do not render the person unable to contain the urine.

Such conditions, however, can become embarrassing when the individual cannot reach the toilet in time. The need to urinate can occur at night, and the older person may face interrupted periods of sleep. Physical accidents are more common at night as persons move about the home in the dark to conserve on electricity. Homes can contain additional environmental hazards by way of loose rugs, sharp-edged furniture, and stairwells.

In older women the pelvic diaphragm, a muscular mass that helps maintain the tone of the bladder and contributes to the proper closure of the bladder outlet, deteriorates. When women age, the pelvic diaphragm becomes weakened, and the bladder does not close completely which leads to leakage or stress incontinence. This can be triggered by coughing or sneezing. Stress incontinence occurs not only in older persons, but in younger individuals, as well. In many cases this can be corrected by retraining and strengthening the muscles.

Dysfunctions

Urinary disorders are a significant cause of death and morbidity within the older population. Total renal functioning is only 50 percent that of young adults. Older persons commonly complain of urinary tract infections, renal complications, and prostate disorders.

There are several symptoms that might signal the start of a urinary disturbance. These include polyuria, nocturia, frequent urination, dysuria, and uremia. Polyuria is a condition characterized by a large volume of urine excreted. It seems to be caused by several factors such as increased fluid intake, diuretics, and disease (i.e., diabetes). Nocturia is defined as the need to urinate during the night, and stems from urinary tract infections, early renal disease, or simply too much fluid intake at night. Dysuria is associated with frequent urination and is usually due to bacterial infection in the urogenital tract. A condition in which blood is found in the normal stream of urine is called hematuria. This is commonly caused by infection, renal problems, and accidents. Finally, uremia, caused by decreased renal blood flow, is a condition in which toxic materials can accumulate in the blood due to the decreased glomerular filtration rate. It is important to note that what is normal and abnormal for individuals varies, but it is considered normal to urinate four to six times daily.

Urinary tract infections have the highest incidence in older people. Ironically, older persons living in private households seem to have the lowest incidence, while persons in hospitals contract these infections at much higher rates.

Infections

Urinary tract infections account for 30-50 percent of all cases of bacteremia and sepsis—a poisoned condition due to the spread of bacteria—in the elderly. Women have traditionally had a higher incidence rate, but there is a gradual increase among men, possibly due to prostate surgery and the presence of bacterial properties in prostate fluid.

Generally the signs of a urinary infection are burning sensations, painful urination, increased nocturnal frequency, suprapubic tenderness, and sometimes fever. Confusion and worsening glucose control in the diabetic may result from such infections.

Cystitis—bacterial infection of the bladder—is common in women with congenitally shorter urethra. Clinical instruments increase the number of infections.

Cystitis is an infection of the urinary bladder, while pyelonephritis or pyelocystitis involve the kidney. Pyelonephritis (or nephritis) is an inflammation of the kidney resulting from recurrent bacterial infections. The condition may become a chronic problem as persons become older causing extensive formation of scar tissue in the kidney. This affects kidney functioning and may cause kidney failure and uremia, a condition in which waste products (urea, creatinine, or uric acid), which are ordinarily excreted, accumulate in the blood. Pyelonephritis generally responds well to treatment with antibiotics. However, it is a serious condition and can cause fatal complications, such as uremia.

There are many factors that play a role in the prevalence of infection among women. Some are the tendency toward having a short urethra in close proximity to the rectal opening, dilation and slowed peristalsis of the urethra and urethral compression by an enlarged uterus during pregnancy. Sociocultural factors also play a role in urinary tract infections. Some are due to the nature of sexual activity, personal hygiene, and socioeconomic status. Diabetes, stones, and gout which are metabolic disturbances appear to lower the system's resistance to infection.

Treatment should begin with a thorough diagnosis to avoid costly and unnecessary therapy. High fluid intake is another part of infective care. It helps relieve symptoms by diluting urine, preventing dehydration, acidifying the urine, and increasing urine flow.

The prostate gland is usually considered the culprit in many urinary tract disorders. The changes in the prostate gland have been divided into two groups: presenile and senile. Presenile occurs between the ages of 40 and 60. It is characterized by irregular change in the smooth muscle fibers and the prostate tissue. The second change, senile, is characterized by a slow and diffuse development, which results in less variation from one part of the gland to another. It occurs between the ages of 60 and 80.

Many older men have prostate problems but do not report symptoms until much later because they may be in denial, and they simply do not want to face the fact that their health is failing. There are three major causes of prostate problems: vesical contracture of the neck, nodular hyperplasia, and carcinoma. Carcinoma of the prostate is rare before the age of 50, but is highly prevalent in men over 80. It commonly spreads to the pelvis and lumbar portion of the spine where it causes great pain. Surgery is usually not recommended because of the advanced state of the condition by the time that it is noted; the surgery would not affect the life expectancy of the person. Some other treatments are radiation therapy, hormonal treatment and radiation of painful metastatic sites. The treatments should be weighed with respect to their side effects. Some men decide not to undergo treatment because they are concerned about their sexual potency.

The urethra, the bladder, the ureter, and the kidney are subject to infection, which is generally more frequent in the elderly. Proper toilet practices and cleansing actions help to prevent infections from gastrointestinal materials.

Prevention can also take the form of increasing fluid intake. Cranberry juice is useful to help destroy bacteria. Sexual practices can play a major role in the development of urinary tract infections; regulating the type or even the frequency of sexual contact can help to prevent or reduce its prevalence. Due to the anatomy of the female, the wiping motion in cleansing, if not done properly, can cause infection. A preventive measure is to initiate wiping with a front to back motion to lessen the risk of spreading bacteria from the anus to the urethral opening.

Kidney Stones

Kidney stones or renal calculi are common between the ages of 30-60. They are more prevalent in men and start in middle-age and increase until old age. These stones are often complications of urinary tract obstructions related to infection and prostate enlargement. Most stones are passed without the use of medical assistance. They are not fatal, but they are very painful, and older persons have a harder time passing these stones. Stones can be prevented through an increased fluid intake. The key to prevention, however, is early diagnosis.

Kidney infections can encourage kidney stone formation by releasing precipitated protein masses and cellular material into the urine, which serve as foci around which the calculi form. Diet and water intake are especially important for bedridden persons since bone demineralization due to inactivity can contribute to increased mineral excretion. Stone formation may also have a genetic component in that urolithiasis tends to occur in families.

Safe substances and procedures are being developed to dissolve or eliminate calculi of certain compositions. Conventional surgery is giving way to sonic fracturing of the calculi by several methods. One technique (lithotripsy) focuses sonic waves on the stones while the patient is in a container of water. Another uses a probe that is surgically placed in the pelvis of the kidney and administers ultrasound energy; in this method, the particles of the stone are rinsed out via the apparatus.

Reasonable dietary practices and adequate water intake adopted as a regular life-style pattern can prevent the formation of kidney stones, even in those who may have inherited a predisposition for them.

Urinary Incontinence

Although urinary incontinence (or involuntary micturition) is a common condition among the elderly, its exact incidence is difficult to establish as it can occur in varying degrees and, in many cases, the person will not admit to being incontinent. Older persons may try to conceal their urinary incontinence because they assume it is due to the aging process, and there is no hope of recovery. They may also be too ashamed and embarrassed to mention it. They may also fear losing their independence and being forced to accept institutional care.

Urinary incontinence is the involuntary loss of urine in undesirable, inappropriate situations. To be continent one must first identify an acceptable place, secondly be able to get there, and thirdly be able to get there in time. It is both a social and health problem, and its incidence increases with age.

In the normal sense incontinence means wetting one's own undergarments or clothes, or, if in bed, the sheets. The incidence of urinary incontinence is more common in women than in men and is usually related to childbirth and weakening of the pelvic floor muscles.

Learning to be continent of urine occurs between 2-5 years of age, and urine is passed approximately 200,000 times in a lifetime. Yet when an accident does occur for the first time, it is treated as a disaster by the person's carers and often by trained health care personnel.

Not surprisingly, the reaction of many elderly people is to keep the problem to themselves and to adapt their lives with various coping strategies. This includes wearing pads, going to the toilet at regular intervals, avoiding going out to strange places, not drinking at certain times of the day and especially at night. Many old people feel incontinence is a normal part of aging and are reluctant to talk to doctors and nurses about this problem.

The bladder is not just a simple balloon which fills from above and drains from below. It has a nerve supply, special lining and musculature known as the detrusor muscle. At the lower end it has an opening known as the sphincter which leads to a passage called the urethra though which urine is passed. Urine reaches the bladder from each kidney through a tube called the ureter. As the bladder fills with urine, a critical volume is reached when the pressure is such that sensory fibers from the stretch receptors are activated and pass a message back to the spinal cord. Nerve centers are then stimulated which give the brain active awareness that the bladder is now full, and, at this time, the desire to pass urine can be overridden. At this point, the individual can walk to a toilet, and the brain can then allow the passing of urine by activating the voiding cycle which causes the detrusor muscle to contract and the sphincter to open. Alternatively, the brain can continue to inform the bladder not to empty. When the capacity fills to a higher level, the sensations are sufficiently uncomfortable to force the person, usually in a hurry, to go to the toilet. If there is further delay, leakage will occur.

In order to be continent, all the nerve pathways have to be intact and the pressure in the urethral sphincter has to be greater than the pressure in the bladder to prevent leakage. The pelvic floor muscles on which the bladder rests have to be strong enough to resist the weight of urine in the bladder and any temporary increase in pressure which occurs with coughing or straining. Leakage under these conditions is known as stress incontinence and even many healthy young women experience it to a small degree.

In an average climate, drinking a normal amount of fluid, the most persons pass is one liter of urine per day and about half a liter of urine at night. People generally pass urine every 2-4 hours during the day and once or twice in the evening. The frequency of passing urine increases both day and night in older people because the bladder has a smaller capacity.

When one wishes to pass urine, the detrusor bladder muscle contracts and the sphincter relaxes to allow voiding. This allows for the passage of urine. In the quiescent phase in between the detrusor muscle does not contract and the sphincter is intact, but, if either or both are malfunctioning, then incontinence or the involuntary passage of urine results.

There are numerous causes which precipitate incontinence, most of which are poorly understood. There are four types of incontinence: stress incontinence, urge incontinence, reflex incontinence, and overflow incontinence.

Stress Incontinence

Stress incontinence involves urine leakage during exercise, coughing, sneezing, or laughing.

In older women weakness of the muscles forming the floor of the pelvic cavity may reduce the effectiveness of the external urethral sphincter. Stress incontinence usually occurs in women especially those whose musculature may have been weakened by multiple vaginal deliveries or pelvic surgery. The pelvic floor muscles help restrict the outlet of the bladder, and their weakness can contribute to leakage of urine from the bladder. It involves the leakage of small amounts of urine with increased abdominal pressure such as that associated with exercise, straining, coughing, laughing or sneezing. Occasionally people who are subject to stress incontinence lose urine when they rise too quickly or change body positions too rapidly.

Urge Incontinence

Urge incontinence is a voluntary urine loss that is immediately preceded by a desire to void.

Urge incontinence involves leakage of varying amounts of urine because of inability to delay voiding before reaching a toilet. It can be, but is not always, caused by a variety of genitourinary and neurological disorders such as involuntary bladder contractions, or local irritation of the bladder or the urethra.

Becoming aware of the need to urinate, which normally is signaled when the bladder is about one-half full, may be delayed in persons over age 65—often until the bladder is almost completely full. Thus, in older persons the need to urinate may be very urgent and, because of weakness of the external urethral sphincter, they may be unable to reach the lavatory in time.

Changes that occur in the kidneys and retention of urine by the bladder make the need to urinate during the night more common in older persons. A significant proportion of elderly people need to wake up to urinate, often several times during the night.

Reflex Incontinence

Reflex incontinence is a sudden loss of large volumes of urine without any sensation of urgency.

Overflow Incontinence

Overflow incontinence consists of a frequent and continuous loss of small amounts of urine with a distended bladder.

There is a higher rate of incontinence among institutionalized older individuals, than those living in the community. Although there is no evidence that normal aging causes incontinence, about 50 percent of older persons in long-term care institutions are incontinent, and approximately 30 percent of all older persons experience some degree of urinary incontinence. This may be, in part, attributable to the fact that persons when they enter long-term care institutions are currently older and sicker. This is, in part, also accounted for by the fact that incontinence is often a cause rather than a result of institutionalization. Furthermore, the incontinence may not have been treated as a resolvable problem and had been allowed to continue unchecked. Programs of water intake and regulating the time of toileting may not have been initiated, nor programs of exercise to strengthen the muscles.

Approximately twice as many women as men suffer from incontinence, and females are less likely to experience a remission. Women are particularly vulnerable to stress incontinence, possibly due to the strain of childbirth which weakens both the bladder outlet and the pelvic muscles. Physically active individuals are less likely to suffer from incontinence. Underlying diseases which can cause incontinence include certain central nervous system disorders such as stroke, multiple sclerosis, diabetes, and Parkinson's disease. Prostatic hypertrophy in men and senile vaginitis in women are other causes. Psychological factors, including attention-seeking, rebellion, regression, and feelings of helplessness and dependency can also contribute to the development of incontinence. Excessive alcohol intake and sedative drugs may be additional contributing factors.

The effects of urinary incontinence on the older person and his or her family are far-reaching. The ability to socialize may be limited. Persons are confined more to their homes. Sooner or later this affects their mental state and morale, and they feel different from or inferior to the rest of society. The home or room can develop an odor, and care of the person can also be an economic burden. Urinary incontinence is, therefore, a common major problem with serious socioeconomic implications.

Incontinence can be psychologically damaging to the individual, and creates aversion in caregivers. Indeed, incontinence is often the reason why institutionalization is sought. Ironically, many institutions will not accept incontinent individuals, indicating a societal reticence in dealing with this problem. Such care, however, can also be quite costly. Incontinence represents a return to an infantile state, returning a previously mature individual to a state of dependency.

Prevention of incontinence is not always possible due to age-related changes and the presence of disease. Encouraging individuals to maintain an active life-style and to participate in appropriate activities can help reduce the incidence of incontinence. Women can often be taught to perform exercises (Kegels) to strengthen the pelvic muscles, or to have surgery to tighten the bladder outlet.

Incontinence is not a normal consequence of aging. Many non-physiological factors are often pertinent to the issue of incontinence. Adequate mental function and motivation must be present for voluntary control of the urinary bladder reflex. The physical ability to move and the skills to do so safely are essential for reaching toilet facilities.

Incontinence should not be accepted as unchangeable or untreatable. In fact, many older individuals are incontinent in the hospital or long-term care setting, but become continent again in their homes, demonstrating the effect of environment on the problem. A positive correlation exists between urinary incontinence and immobility.

Postmenopausal women experience atrophy of the musculature in the bladder sphincters, lessened tone of the urethral smooth muscle, atrophic vaginitis (regression and inflammation of the vagina), and weakening of other muscles of the pelvic floor. These changes are related to trauma to the area from childbirth or surgery as well as to the cessation of estrogen production that characterizes menopause. The fact that the female urethra is much shorter than the male's may add to the likelihood that urinary control can be easily lost. Estrogen replacement therapy and specific exercises for pelvic muscles are useful.

There are many emotional issues linked to urinary incontinence and involve issues of self-esteem. The onset of urinary incontinence can lead to social withdrawal, and can serve to promote mental and physical health problems. To be incontinent is not an image that most persons entertain of themselves.

Emotional factors also seem to be involved in some instances of incontinence. Older persons can manipulate caregivers by becoming incontinent and can enlist the attention of children.

Nocturia

Nocturia, or excessive urination at night, is a common problem. People using prescription drugs or who have several chronic diseases frequently have to wake several times a night to urinate. Having to urinate several times at night is a disturbance of sleep and may pose additional problems for persons who have sleep difficulties.

It is particularly important for older persons to have periods of undisturbed rest at night to offset the deleterious effects of stress. Noisy home or institutional environments can be disturbing. General health can be markedly affected by inadequate rest and sleep.

It is also important for older persons to completely empty the bladder upon urination. A total depletion of the bladder is important so that residual urine does not remain and cause the older person to experience urine spills after just having left the toilet.

Urinary incontinence is often the precipitating cause for placing an older individual in a nursing home. The inconvenience and the work associated in caring for an incontinent older person leads to this decision. There are incontinence programs which, if proper community assistance is available, can allow the family to maintain the person at home. Assistance by way of confidential laundry service, water ingestion regimens and timing of when the person will need to void, all are important alternatives to institutionalization based on incontinence.

An environmental inventory of the home and the barriers that may be present in the home that serve as obstacles to reaching the bathroom within the needed time, is very helpful. Adequate nighttime lighting, non-slip rugs, and paperless toilets are all important aids in keeping the person continent. Such considerations are particularly important when persons suffer from chronic diseases which lead to frequent urination, such as diabetes.

Dysfunctions Caused by the Prostate Gland

Thousands of men yearly face the problem of prostatic enlargement, with the symptoms of painful urination, difficult urination, urine retention, infection and tenderness. In those afflicted, prostatitis may occur as early as the late 40s to early 50s. Regular examinations are important for early detection of the problem.

While the prostate gland is an organ of the reproductive system, it can also frequently interfere with the functioning of the urinary system of older men. The prostate gland is located very near the opening from the male bladder. It has, literally lying on it, the urethra, a tube used to drain the bladder. When the prostate is enlarged or swollen, the pressure on the urethra interferes with the normal flow of urine. Urination becomes difficult, and the bladder is never completely emptied. There is an overall atrophy of the prostate with aging; however, a significant number of men over the age of 60 experience nodular growths (hyperplasia) in their prostate. This often interferes with the free flow of urine.

The main function of the prostate is to produce the seminal fluid which acts as a vehicle for the delivery of sperm. Without these fluids, the male becomes sterile, although his libido is not necessarily affected. On the other hand, the male with prostate problems often has serious problems with his sex life, primarily because of the urine retention situation and possible low-grade infection. Appropriate nutrition, in combination with a dietary and exercise support program, can help to promote healthy prostate function.

In benign hyperplasia of the prostate gland, men experience reduced force behind their stream of urine. Men who suffer from this disease also urinate frequently, are unable to empty their bladders completely, and may dribble after urination. Enlargement of the prostate may be surgically corrected. The procedure is called transurethral resection. An instrument is passed up the urethra, and the portion of the gland compressing the urethra is removed.

The most common tumor found in older men is carcinoma of the prostate. It affects approximately 50 percent of the men over the age of 70. Only one-third of these cancers, however, become clinically significant.

Initially, a prostatic tumor may cause little or no urethral obstruction. Thus,in the early stages, a person may be aware of the tumor. When the tumor enlarges to the point where it interferes with the flow of urine, the condition may be too advanced for effective treatment. As preventive measures, older men should have routine prostate gland examinations. Since blood levels of a particular protein are usually elevated, a blood test called the prostate-specific antigen (PSA) test that indicates the presence of this protein is a common procedure, along with a digital rectal examination. If not detected early, the cancer may spread from the prostate gland to other areas. In some instance, drug therapy may produce remissions of some duration. Surgical removal is generally the most successful treatment for carcinoma of the prostate.

Technology in Diagnosis and Treatment

New technology has been applied to help remedy some of the problems caused by diseases of the urinary system. Measurements of kidney function allow more accurate diagnosis, and certain technical aids can help compensate for the loss of function.

Renal Dialysis and Transplant

The most dramatic methods that are used to accommodate an individual's need for kidney function during and after renal failure are renal dialysis (the artificial kidney) and kidney transplant. Renal dialysis has been in use long enough to be considered effective in augmenting kidney function. In dialysis, toxic materials are removed as would occcur in a normally functioning kidney.

The role of the kidney as an endocrine organ is lost if it is missing or destroyed by disease. One such hormone called erythropoietin stimulates red blood cell production. Without it, anemias (lack of red blood cells) will result. This can lead to a variety of additional medical problems. The availability of commercially produced erythropoietin offsets this loss to a large extent.

Kidney transplantation is also a successful treatment method for end-stage renal disease (ESRD). The ability to determine the cellular antigens of prospective donors and recipients has made it possible to match them closely, significantly reducing immunological rejection. Also, the availability of dialysis and the slower onset of dysfunction in chronic renal failure allows more time to search for appropriate donors than is the case with other organ transplants. Finally, newer agents to control the immunological rejection of foreign tissue have improved survival of grafts with less severe side effects for the recipient. If a living donor and recipient are "complete" tissue matches, graft survival for two years is nearly 100 percent. If careful "partial" matches are made with a living donor, the survival is nearly as good. Even kidneys taken in a timely manner from cadavers (persons who have already died) survive two or more years in their hosts 75 percent of the time or longer. The transplanted kidney may restore normal endocrine function related to blood pressure control and active vitamin D production.

The suitability of older persons as either recipients or donors of kidneys is an important issue. The diminished capacity of the older kidney due to glomerular attrition makes its use for transplantation questionable, even after death. In addition, an older living donor, left with a single, older kidney, may not be able to manage.

Renal Replacement Therapy in Older Persons

The elderly were frequently excluded from early dialysis programs. With the increasing availability of dialysis, particularly throughout the United States, these patients are now admitted to the program.

Some studies suggest that older patients on hemodialysis do as well as younger ones. Older patients are often more compliant with diet and medication regimens. However, care of the elderly requires special considerations. Older patients suffer from a variety of medical problems at the same time. There is also a high first-year mortality rate among older patients.

Renal Calculi

Although renal calculi, or kidney stones, are more common in younger persons, the presence of stones in the urinary bladder does become progressively more common with aging. If a stone becomes lodged within the ureter, it may obstruct the flow of urine to the bladder, causing it to build up within the renal pelvis and eventually damaging the kidney. Kidney stones are particularly serious in older persons because they have more difficulty passing them than do younger persons. Advances in laser treatments and surgery can considerably lessen the dangers of this condition.

In general, the most serious danger to the functioning of the urinary system derives from the number and types of medications employed in treatment procedures. Because older persons often suffer from as many as three or more chronic ailments at the same time, their treatments include high levels of drug dosages.

Interventions and Technology

Many technologies are specific to a particular type or types of incontinence and attempt to cure the problem (e.g., artificial sphincters, electric stimulators, drugs, training procedures, and surgery). Diagnostic evaluation is thus critical to the appropriate use of these treatments. Other treatment technologies are non-specific and palliative rather than curative (bedpads, undergarments and, in some situation, catheters). In general, these technologies should be used as a last resort after diagnostic evaluation has excluded treatable conditions.

The various types of technologies for the treatment of urinary incontinence fall into approximately four categories: devices, surgery, drug treatment, and training procedures.

Examples of devices include catheters to collect urine before leakage occurs. A flexible tube is placed directly in the bladder and drains urine into a collecting bag. Catheters can be used continually or intermittently. The use of catheters is recommended when there exists the inability to empty the bladder (urinary retention) which cannot be corrected by surgical or drug treatment. The danger of infection must be carefully controlled.

Devices to prevent or delay urine outflow include the artificial sphincters which consist of an inflatable cuff which is surgically implanted around the urethra and inflated to prevent urine outflow. For females, electrical stimulation through a device inserted into the vagina produces electric impulses that cause contraction of pelvic floor musculature and inhibits bladder contractions. For males, an external penis clamp can be used to prevent urine flow.

Four major types of devices are currently in use: bedpads and undergarments, catheters, electrical stimulation, and artificial sphincters.

Bedpads and undergarments range from those that are completely disposable to those with launderable components. Most acute care hospitals and long-term care institutions use "blue pads" for managing incontinence despite their relatively low absorbency and lack of odor control. More innovative forms, like the Kylie(C) pad that is launderable and draws moisture away from the body, have been marketed widely in the United States only recently. The efficacy of these products in diminishing complications of incontinence such as skin irritation and urinary tract infection has not yet been carefully assessed.

The three types of catheters commonly used are chronic indwelling catheters, intermittent bladder catheterization, and, for men, external catheters. A Foley indwelling catheter is placed in the bladder and attached to plastic tubing that drains urine into an externally worn collection bag. This type of catheter can induce serious complications, however; urinary tract infection is the most common. It should only be used in patients with urinary retention that cannot be treated surgically, pharmacologically, or by intermittent catheterization, and for patients with skin conditions that are worsened by contact with urine.

External (condom) catheters, used exclusively in men, may reduce infection but require frequent changing, often fall off, and may result in local skin irritation. The National Aeronautics and Space Administration (NASA) has also developed an external female urine-collection device for use of women astronauts. This device may be appropriate for use with some patients.

Electrical stimulation involves an external device that intermittently stimulates musculature associated with voiding to induce muscle contraction and maintain continence. This technique is most useful for incontinence due to stress and bladder instability.

Devices to Correct Urinary Incontinence

Incontinence is a symptom with many possible causes. As a symptom, it requires full investigation to establish the diagnosis, followed by specific treatment with drugs, physiotherapy, or surgery. External devices should be considered only if these treatments are ineffective. However, many elderly patients with chronic incontinence suffer from a degree of mental impairment limiting their tolerance of certain external devices.

A high percentage of stroke victims and victims of Parkinsonism suffer from some degree of incontinence. Incontinence associated with dementia, a deterioration of intellectual abilities, may be a result of direct involvement of those areas of the brain involved in bladder control, or it may be secondary to the patient's inattention to personal hygiene, inability to communicate needs to the nursing staff, or inability to reach the toilet. Urinary incontinence continues to escalate as a problem in long-term care facilities as the age of admission increases, along with the numbers of persons with multiple severe diseases.

Restoration of urinary control has included application of implantable, indwelling, and external devices. Both electrical and mechanical technologies have been utilized.

Despite severe drawbacks, an indwelling catheter and a diaper or pad are the two most widely employed devices for managing urinary incontinence. Their ease of application and their ability to control leakage in the case of the catheter or to provide storage in the case of the pad, as well as lack of suitable alternative management schemes, have encouraged their widespread use.

The indwelling catheter allows for continuous bladder draining in seriously disabled and totally incontinent patients, requires less attention than intermittent types of incontinence care, and does not require patient capability. The indwelling catheter may be indicated as the method of care for a patient who is senile or bedridden, or who has upper-body disabilities that make self-care impossible.

The drawbacks of the indwelling catheter are several: the patient's mobility is severely limited; the incidence of urinary tract and bladder infection and irritation is extremely high; and, the catheter requires changing by professional staff. Bacteria will eventually develop in virtually all cases.

The use of a diaper or pad will allow patient mobility, and can be an aid in the management of incontinence of the bowel, as well as of the bladder. Problems with this type of care include skin irritation, the need for frequent changes to ensure local hygiene, an unpleasant odor, infections of the urinary tract, and the psychological stigma of wearing a diaper. Such garments are available in a variety of sizes, geared to the nature of the urinary problem. Some of these undergarments are treated with absorbent substances that absorb much of the urine, preventing discomfort and skin diseases.

Because of these drawbacks to the use of indwelling catheters and diapers or pads, alternative device treatment modalities, including surgically implanted devices and external patient-applied methods, have been developed.

REFERENCES

Hampton, J.K., Craven, R.F., & Heitkemper, M.M. (1997). *The Biology of Human Aging* (2nd ed.). Dubuque, IA: Wm. C. Brown.

Harris, R. (Ed.). (1983). *Medical devices and instrumentation for the elderly.* Arlington, VA: Association for the Advancement of Medical Instrumentation.

Kart, S. K., Metress, E. K., & Metress, S. P. (1992). *Human Aging and Chronic Disease.* Boston: Jones & Bartlett.

Lesnoff-Caravaglia, G. (Ed.). (1987). *Handbook of Applied Gerontology.* New York: Human Sciences Press.

Oram, J.J. (1997). *Caring for the Fourth Age.* London: Armelle.

Spence, D.A. (1995). *The Biology of Human Aging* (2nd ed.). Englewood Cliffs, NJ: Prentice-Hall.

Technology and Aging in America. (1985). (OTA-BA-264). Washington, DC: U.S. Congress, Office of Technology Assessment.

Chapter 9

THE REPRODUCTIVE SYSTEM

The sexuality of older persons has not been freely or openly discussed until recently. The topic of sex, in general, was not discussed in an easy or comfortable framework. One reason why society now refers more openly to sex is due to the increasing numbers of older persons who, by living beyond the period of procreation, have linked sex, not to reproduction of the species, but to pleasure.

Increases in life expectancy have led to the survival of the species long after childbearing and child rearing ages and has led to a greater interest in sex as a pleasurable and socially fulfilling activity. It is no longer sex for procreation, but sex as recreation. This change is due, in part, to more sophisticated methods of contraception, but also in part to the increasing numbers of older persons within the population.

The concept of sex as pleasure and personal fulfillment rose as the aging population increased. Sex linked solely to reproduction became an anachronism. The life expectancy for women has increased, and large numbers of women are living beyond menopause. This means that the years of life experienced by a woman after menopause may be greater than her sexually reproductive years. Alterations in demography which leave more older women than men to experience life to advanced ages, also means that fewer men are available as sexual partners. This older population represents individuals who were married, widowed, divorced, or never-married; all of whom had a decided interest in maintaining continuity in their lives–including sexual continuity.

The concept of living with another person to whom one was not married was not introduced by younger persons, but, rather, by the increasing presence of an older population. For varying reasons, personal, economical, familial, or societal, older persons found it more convenient not to contract formal marriages. Social Security laws which advantaged single persons over married ones also promoted such choices. Many adult children, however, spend anguished hours attempting to reconcile a parent's new life-style.

The financial stability experienced by many older persons which permits them to travel and to lead active social lives contributes to the expansion of their interpersonal interests. It was once commonplace for women to think that once their reproductive life was over, life itself was over. In the traditional model, the purpose of a woman's life was to marry, care for her husband, bear children, and to finally act as nurse to her ailing aged spouse. Few women would today subscribe to such a notion.

Movements such as the Women's Liberation were long loath to include older women as part of their agenda. The negative stereotyping of older women prevailed even in these circles. Their inclusion in such groups was the product of efforts of older female activists, some of whom formed their own organizations. Their gradual acceptance by such groups was due largely to the simple preponderance of older women in society.

Sexuality and Intimacy

Intimacy is perhaps a more appropriate term to use in describing the sexual interests of some older persons. They may not engage in coitus, but experience a great deal of satisfaction from the presence of a person, and through fondling, embracing or kissing. Just being simply linked in the minds of other persons to another human being in a very personal way is sexually satisfying. This sense of belonging has very positive physical and psychological benefits. The need to belong, the need to love, is as real in old age as at any other age level. The need to love someone, as well as the need to be loved in return, is a basic human need that transcends age.

Contributing to the difficulty of openly recognizing the sexuality of older persons lies in the fact that children generally considered their parents to be sexless individuals. Many women would have great difficulty in discussing a sexual problem with an adult daughter. Remarriage for older men and women was problematic largely due to the attitudes of children. The fact that most older men are married or are few in number, causes most older women to become sexually deprived. Since physical changes are not extensive in old age with respect to the reproductive system, older persons, barring poor health, can continue to be sexually active indefinitely.

The reproductive system plays an important role in the lives of older persons. Negative stereotyping of older individuals and a negative attitude towards sexuality in old age has delayed scientific research in this area of human experiencing. The reproductive system does not sustain extensive physiological changes, but those that may occur are felt more on an emotional or psychological level. Changes in the reproductive system have a significant bearing on personal identity and self concept. Alterations in sexual functioning, more than any other bodily system, may signify to the person that he or she is old. For men, erectile dysfunction can undermine physical and mental well-being. One of the major physiological changes in women is menopause with its concomitant hormonal changes which can result in physical and psychological consequences such as mood alterations, irritability, and depression. Not all women experience such changes to the same degree, and some experience menopause with equanimity.

Physiological Changes in Males

There are physiological changes that affect the sexual functioning of older males. The testes decrease in size and firmness with age. There is a gradual decline in the secretion of testosterone. The decline in testosterone levels in the blood may reduce muscle strength and sperm production. It also contributes to the general wasting appearance of older men.

Older men generally experience reduced sexual desires which may be the result of lower testosterone levels. Since men are more prone to premature aging due to life-style and vocational hazards, this may also play a role in, not only lower testosterone levels, but in the susceptibility to diseases in old age. Also, as they age, men who suffer from disabilities or illnesses are less likely to be sexually active.

The capability to engage in intercourse can continue into advanced old age. Sperm production continues into old age, but there is a decline in the number of sperm and in their motility after approximately the age of 50. There may be adequate numbers of viable sperm in the semen of octogenarians and nonagenarians to make fertilization possible. There are recorded instances of centenarians fathering children.

Men do not experience a major physiological change such as the menopause experienced by women. Many men do, however, exhibit a form of panic behavior sometimes referred to as the "male menopause," which has more psychological features than physical. Men view with dismay their graying hair and increased weight, and fear that their professional, occupational, or sexual opportunities may have begun to shrink. They may undergo an identity crisis. Such panic may also manifest itself in increased sexual activity, the engaging in extra-marital affairs, and the adoption of behavior that simulates the actions of younger men. Such changes include a more youthful dress, increase in alcohol consumption, increase in tobacco or drug use, and the display of a form of exhibitionism which calls attention to their masculinity. Although such behavior is not necessarily manifest in all men, such reactions often occur in men at reaching the ages of 45 or 50. A common picture of such behavior is a man in his fifties, driving an ostentatious convertible sports car, dressed in expensive designer sport clothes, with a very young blonde female at his side.

The eruption of such behaviors often disrupts family life, results in divorce, and creates divisive families. Many of the financial and social problems faced by older females are the result of such male mid-life crises. The loss of an ordered family life and a support group often has bitter echoes for males in old age. Estranged children find it difficult to be concerned about or to provide care for an aged parent who abandoned them in their youth. There are men, however, who do successfully establish second and third families during their lifetimes.

Such behavioral changes are very likely related to reductions in testosterone levels. Although physiologically such changes are not as dramatic as is menopause for females, the psychosocial effects can be as far-reaching.

Additional physiological changes include reductions in the volume of fluid contributed to semen by the prostate, and the force behind its contraction during orgasm. The prostate gland surrounding the urethra frequently enlarges with age. The gland may double in weight by the time a male reaches the age of 70.

The penis tends to become smaller. After approximately age 55, the walls of the blood vessels and the erectile tissue in the penis become somewhat rigid and less elastic. The older male is slower to achieve an erection, and it is likely to be less firm. Such losses of elasticity can prevent the attainment of an erection. Older males are less likely to experience sexual stimulation from visual stimuli and may require more direct stimulation. They may also have an intermittent loss of ejaculatory ability. This may also lead to a decrease in the expulsive force of the seminal fluid. Nonetheless, even at advanced ages, men are usually capable of satisfying sexual relationships.

The common changes in the male reproductive system cause some men to become depressed, to experience mood swings, or to become aware of their own finitude. The advent of old age is a precursor of death. The prospect of growing old is viewed with trepidation, alarm, and sometimes fear. Psychosocial factors play a large role in attitudes toward self and sexual activity. The first experience of impotence can provoke much self-reflection and anxiety.

Physiological Changes in Females

Changes in sexual activity among women are related more to the absence of available men in the older population. Also, older men tend more to select younger women as sexual partners. This is due in part to the societal view that older women are less attractive and desirable, and that sex is more appropriately engaged in by the younger population.

The recent trend for older women to marry younger men is probably more true of wealthier and more privileged population groups. There is, however, greater acceptance of such couples, particularly when it is a second or third marriage. The rise in multiple marriages and in the number of people who simply live together has also served to blur age differences.

Physiological changes in the female reproductive system appear initially in the ovaries, resulting in the production of reduced amounts of estrogens and progesterone. The diminishing hormonal levels cause degenerative changes in the vagina, uterus, and in the external genitalia. The level of estrogens in the blood does not alter until about age 40. After this age, there is a gradual decline until the age of 60 when it becomes stabilized.

The low level of estrogens results in the cessation of the menstrual cycle. Menopause usually occurs in women in their 40s or 50s, but can initiate in the 60s. The hormonal changes occur gradually over a period of time. There is reduction in menstrual flow, and, eventually, the spacing between menstrual periods is increased. Following menopause, the adrenal glands are the primary source of estrogens in postmenopausal women.

At the onset of menopause, women can experience a variety of physical and psychological changes. Some women are subject to hot flashes, sweating, or red blotches on the face and chest. Others become emotionally labile with periods of depression or irritability. Somatic complaints such as headache, nervousness, and insomnia are common. Sensory losses may be accentuated, such as vision. Problems in dental care may surface. Many women, however, experience this major physiological change with few or none of these symptoms. For some, it is a source of relief—a form of freedom from biological entrapment.

For some women the psychological effects of menopause are more telling. The fact that a woman cannot conceive or have any more children can bring on depressive states and questions of self-identity and a sense of loss of femininity. Because they are no longer menstruating, some feel that they are now indeed old, and they may see themselves as unattractive and uninteresting, reinforcing the negative stereotype of older women. Weight gain and loss of interest in personal appearance can also result.

For others, menopause spells freedom from a biological function. Since there is no longer the fear of pregnancy, some women feel free to increase their sexual activity. Unfortunately, many older women are unaware of the fact that they can contract AIDS if they do not practice safe sex. Since they can no longer become pregnant, they tend not to use precautions related to the transmission of sexually transmitted diseases.

Older women may also experience some masculinizing changes which include a change in voice level, with some women developing deeper, lower voices. This is truer of women whose life-style includes smoking and the consumption of alcohol. Other physical changes include an increase in facial hair such as a beard or moustache. Some women have a hereditary tendency toward baldness, and this may occur as rapidly thinning hair or actual bald spots. The chin may appear to be more prominent, especially if there are changes in dental structure. Women who are edentulous develop the profile characteristic of the Halloween witch. Many such physical changes can all be altered by cosmetic interventions. Plastic surgery is often practiced in ambulatory care centers and, as their use and acceptance has increased, such interventions have become increasingly affordable. It is conceivable that the ability to alter physical appearance is without limits. Some bodily changes can be effected through appropriate exercise regimens and diet.

In women the reproductive system undergoes various structural changes. The vagina becomes shorter, and loses width and elasticity. It also changes color from a reddish purple to a light pink. Its walls become thin. Glands that lubricate the vagina atrophy, and the vagina becomes dry. As a result, sexual intercourse can become difficult or painful. Such changes can be corrected through physical therapy. Due to diminished levels of estrogens, there may be a delayed sense of arousal, and the number and intensity of orgasms may be reduced.

The vaginal secretions are less acidic in postmenopausal women, allowing for the growth of bacteria and yeasts. As a result, vaginal infections can potentially increase.

Interest in sexual activity and the ability to engage in satisfying intercourse do not decline in older women. The frequency of intercourse for older women is often compromised by lack of a partner due to widowhood or divorce. The health and sexual capacities of partners may be considerably diminished due to disease or physical handicaps. Such factors can seriously erode an older woman's sexual activity.

Hormonal decline following menopause causes changes in the structure of the female body and the external genitalia. Women tend to gain fat in areas such as the waist, thighs, and buttocks. The skin develops wrinkles and hangs in folds. Hair is spread more sparsely over the body, the scalp, and the pubic area. The clitoris reduces in size. The genital labia become thinner, lose color, and are less prominent. The breasts are less firm, and the nipples may decrease in size and sensitivity.

Dysfunctions

Cancer

One dysfunction of the reproductive system that is more prevalent with age is cancer. Older men frequently experience cancer of the prostate. The incidence of cancer of the ovary, uterus, vagina, cervix, and breast is greater in postmenopausal women.

Older persons require regular examinations to detect symptoms of cancer. Men should have their prostate gland palpated each year. Women should seek pelvic examinations and have mammograms when indicated. Self-examination of the breasts should be conducted routinely. Vaginal bleeding or spotting should receive medical attention.

Breast cancer is a problem for approximately 1 out of every 12 women in the United States. Risk factors for developing breast cancer include factors such as age and family history.

Breast examination is important in older women in whom the incidence of breast cancer is higher. About 40 percent of women with breast cancer are aged 70 or older. Giving women of 70 or over appropriate treatment can enable them to reach a five-year survival rate similar to that for younger women. There are probably multifactorial reasons why doctors do not routinely perform breast examinations: some feel uncomfortable, a few lack confidence, and some are deterred by claims of assault. Some physicians do not like to touch older persons, and many older women during physical checkups are not given breast examinations.

Early detection is the best protection against breast cancer. Mammography is capable of detecting a breast tumor while it is still too small to be noticeable by self-examination.

Atrophic Vaginitis

Changes occur in the lining of the female reproductive tract that lead to inflammation of the vagina. Such changes are principally due to the reduced level of estrogens in the postmenopausal woman. When the inflammation is linked to degenerative changes, the condition is known as atrophic vaginitis.

In postmenopausal women, the walls of the vagina are thinner and less moist. Consequently, they are more easily damaged. Such damaged surfaces, in the process of healing, may grow together, thus closing off the vaginal canal.

In older women, vaginal acidic secretions are reduced. Reduced acidic secretions permit the growth of protozoans, yeasts, and bacteria which are conducive to inflammations.

Prolapse of the Uterus

A common dysfunction of the reproductive system is prolapse of the uterus. This condition results when the ligaments become too weak to support the organ. The uterus drops through the cervical canal and then protrudes into the vagina. Damages experienced during childbirth can contribute to this condition. This problem also occurs in women who do not exercise sufficiently, or who are bedridden, and in women in advanced old age who have not engaged in sexual activity over a prolonged period of time.

The utilization of a pessary in the vagina helps to correct this problem. Surgical intervention is also a possibility.

Erectile Dysfunction

The term "impotence" has been traditionally used to signify the inability of the male to attain and maintain erection of the penis sufficient to permit satisfactory sexual intercourse. It is recommended that the more precise term "erectile dysfunction" be used instead to signify an inability of the male to achieve an erect penis as part of the overall multifaceted process of male sexual function.

Erectile dysfunction affects millions of men. This condition is not necessarily age-related, but it is progressively more frequent as men become older. Men who suffer from a variety of physical ailments may be prone to such dysfunctions, particularly diabetics. This is a problem among men who consume large quantities of alcohol, have cardiovascular problems, or are habitual users of drugs for medical reasons or as recreation. Stress and emotional or psychological problems are additional factors that can lead to erectile dysfunction. Counseling and medical intervention can assist in dealing with particular life-style problems or psychological problems.

Erectile dysfunction is often incorrectly assumed to be a natural concomitant of the aging process. In older men, erectile dysfunction may occur as a consequence of specific illnesses such as diabetes mellitus, or of medical treatment for certain illnesses. It can result in fear, loss of image and self-confidence, and depression. Furthermore, the embarrassment experienced by older men in discussing sexual issues and the discomfort of health care providers in dealing with this problem, creates a climate unfavorable for pursuing treatment.

There is scarce information on the variations in prevalence of erectile dysfunction across geographic, racial, ethnic, socioeconomic, and cultural groups. In males of all ages, erectile failure may discourage initiating sexual relationships because of fear of inadequate sexual performance or rejection. Older males are particularly sensitive to the social support of intimate relationships. To have to withdraw from such relationships, when other coping capabilities are also in jeopardy, can have a negative effect on overall health.

Erectile dysfunction can be caused by a number of factors, including physical disorders of the vascular or nervous systems, diabetes, prostate surgery, excessive alcohol, high blood cholesterol levels, lack of sexual knowledge, poor sexual techniques, inadequate interpersonal relationships or their deterioration, and many chronic diseases, especially renal failure and dialysis. Smoking has an adverse effect on erectile function by accentuating the effects of other risk factors such as vascular disease or hypertension. A number of medications, particularly those taken to lower blood pressure, can also be a risk factor. A certain percentage of the cases may be psychological in nature, and counseling is often beneficial.

Some cases of impotence can be treated by vascular surgery. Penile implants are utilized with greater frequency. There are three forms of penile prostheses available: semirigid, malleable, and inflatable. A flexible rod or an inflatable cylinder is surgically implanted in the penis to provide the rigidity necessary for sexual intercourse. Penile prostheses are indicated only for carefully selected patients.

The development of the drug Viagra® has been helpful to counter the problem in many instances. The drug, sildenafil citrate, is taken about an hour before intercourse and was found in studies to help 70 percent to 80 percent of impotent subjects. It acts on the normal physiological system in the penis and elicits an erection when a man is sexually stimulated; it has no effect if he is not.

Erectile dysfunction affects half of all men between the ages of 40 and 70, resulting in problems of getting or maintaining an erection. Reticence in discussing this sexual problem causes fewer than 10 percent of impotent men to actively seek treatment.

Erectile dysfunction can be effectively treated with a variety of methods. Many patients and health care providers are unaware of these treatments, and the dysfunction thus often remains untreated, compounded by its psychological impact.

Diminished Sexual Functioning

In general, there is a decrease in sexual activity as persons grow older. This is true of males and females, although there is less of a decline for females. The onset of such decline differs for males and females, with a decline beginning after their twenties for males and much later for females.

Physiological changes that occur in the body may alter the ability to perform or to derive pleasure from sexual activity. In the female, there is a decrease in the amount of blood flow to the breasts, labia, and clitoris, which are all areas highly sensitive to touch. With this decrease in vascularization, there is less of a stimulus response, and thus less pleasure may be derived, or it may take longer to become aroused. It takes longer for an older woman to reach orgasm; orgasms may be reduced in number and intensity. It also takes longer for the vagina to be lubricated during the excitatory phase which may cause an increase in friction during intercourse leading to discomfort or pain. The decrease in the width and length of the vagina and uterus can add further discomfort. The muscles surrounding the pubic area and outer part of the vagina can involuntarily contract and cramp as a protective response, causing additional pain. This condition is known as vaginismus.

For males, there is usually a decrease in the firmness of the erection, and it takes longer to develop. Males experience less need to ejaculate. Some of these symptoms may be due to the fact that the person is taking antidepressant drugs or antipsychotic drugs, which have a tendency to impair one's ability to have an erection. Sexual dysfunction can also result from vascular diseases which decrease the amount of blood flow to the penis. Diabetes and nutrition can play a role in sexual dysfunction.

Diminished sexual functioning can be dependent upon additional factors, such as mental health or alterations in physical appearance. As people age, they frequently gain weight and may feel that they are no longer attractive or aesthetically pleasing.

Boredom with a partner of some 50 years may also lead to a disinterest in sex. With the increase in life expectancy, marriages can last for much longer. This may also account for the increase in divorce rates among persons over the age of 65.

The negative stereotypical view that sex is the province of the young can lead some older persons to view their interest in sex as improper, immoral, or abnormal. Women had long been expected to remain true to their dead husbands, and the physical death of the husband led to the social death of the surviving widow.

Nutritional deficiencies such as decreased zinc or increased caffeine also have an effect upon sexual functioning. Alcohol also interferes with proper sexual functioning. Extended abstinence can also render it more difficult to resume normal functioning at a later period.

By and large, older persons can continue satisfying sexual lives into advanced old age. For most persons, it is not the physiological ability to perform or the absence of interest in sexual activity, but rather the unavailability of a sexual partner. The sexual deprivation experienced by older women can lead to depression and social withdrawal. The importance of sexual expression is becoming increasingly recognized as society moves further and further from the notion of sex as procreation. Sexuality is a social, psychological and physical problem.

Technology and Sexuality

Assistive Insemination

Assistive insemination has radically altered the possibilities of reproduction in older women, even after menopause. Whereas it was possible for older men to have families at advanced ages, it is now possible for postmenopausal women to bear children. This can mean that women, along with men, can now have second and third families. Being able to procreate in old age suggests that women can biologically have the same sexual capabilities as men. In terms of the reproductive system, age may indeed become irrelevant.

Women in their 60s have borne healthy children, and older women continue to express interest in becoming parents at advanced ages. Some women bear children for other infertile family members or provide children to childless couples. The capability to be able to "rent a womb" extends now to the older female as well.

In assistive insemination, the sperm can be supplied by the husband, and the egg from a donor. The older mother carries the fetus to term and becomes the gestating mother. In some instances, both the sperm and the egg are donated.

Further, women can at younger ages freeze and save their own eggs for use in assistive insemination when they are postmenopausal. An older couple, for example, can utilize both the husband's sperm and the wife's egg to form a new family related to their older children who can be several decades apart in age.

Some nations have attempted to halt the birth of children to older mothers because there is the fear that she may not live long enough to nurture the child. In cases where the father has been over 70, there has not been a similar outcry.

REFERENCES

Chop, W. C. & Robnett, R. H. (1999). *Gerontology for the Health Care Professional.* Philadelphia: F.A. Davis Company.

DiGovanna, A. G. (1994). *Human Aging.* New York: McGraw-Hill, Inc.

Freedman, A., Hahn, G. & Love, N. (1996). Follow-up after therapy for prostate cancer. *Postgraduate Medicine, 100*(3), 125-134.

Godschalk, M., Sison, A., & Mulligan, T. (1997). Management of erectile dysfunction by the geriatrician. *JAGS,45*(10), 1240-1246.

Kart, C. S. (1997). *The Realities of Aging.* Boston: Allyn and Bacon.

Kart, C. S., Metress, E. K., & Metress, S. P. (1992). *Human Aging and Chronic Disease.* Boston: Jones & Bartlett.

Lesnoff-Caravaglia, G. (1987). *Handbook of Applied Gerontology.* New York: Human Sciences Press.

Oram, J. J. (1997). *Caring for the Fourth Age.* London: Armelle Press.

Rowe, J. W., & Kahn, R. L. *Successful Aging.* (1998). New York: Pantheon.

Schulz, R., & Salthouse, T. (Eds.). (1995). *Adult Development and Aging* (3rd ed.). Upper Saddle River, NJ: Prentice-Hall.

Schneider, E. L., & Rose, J.W. (Eds.). (1990). *Handbook of the Biology of Aging* (3rd ed.). New York: Academic Press.

Spence, A.P. (1995). *Biology of Human Aging.* Englewood Cliffs, NJ: Prentice Hall.

Taub, M., Begas, A., & Love, N. (1996). Advanced prostate cancer. *Postgraduate Medicine, 100*(3), 139-154.

Chapter 10

THE ENDOCRINE AND IMMUNE SYSTEMS

THE ENDOCRINE SYSTEM

The endocrine system is poorly understood, although its vital connection to other body systems is clear. It is this system that is responsible for homeostasis. Much like the nervous system, the endocrine system is one of the main regulatory systems of the body.

It helps regulate body temperature, basal metabolic rate, growth rate, stress responses, and reproductive functions.

The endocrine system is made up of glands that work closely with the nervous system to maintain internal body balance and stable conditions. The glands control a number of body processes by way of hormones that are directed toward specific organs throughout the body. Endocrine glands include the pituitary or the master gland, the thyroid, the parathyroids, the adrenals, the pancreas, and the gonads. The hypothalamus region of the brain is also linked to endocrine functions. The hypothalamus is also considered as possibly the site of an "aging clock" that controls the aging process.

The hormones excreted by these glands play very important roles in areas such as sexual identity and activity and the development of secondary sexual characteristics. The hormones are specialized in that they are targeted for specific cells. Hormonal imbalances can induce far-reaching bodily changes, including extremes such as dwarfism and gigantism. The aging process itself may be the result of a programmed deficiency of one or more hormones. The aging process could possibly be manipulated through the addition of hormones and hormone-secreting cells.

The ability of endocrine glands to synthesize hormones does not decrease to a great extent as persons age. However, the role of the pituitary gland in regulating growth has led to speculation that the maintaining of levels of growth hormone might slow the rate of aging.

Dysfunctions

The endocrine system does not present many difficulties as persons age. Pathological changes, rather than those due to the process of aging, are more likely to be the cause of a disorder. The activity of the endocrine glands is closely interrelated, and a single disturbance can have wide-ranging effects. This is also due to its connections to the nervous system. In older persons, endocrine dysfunction can result in diabetes mellitus, stress reactions, and hypothyroidism (goiters).

Diabetes Mellitus

Persons can inherit a predisposition toward diabetes, and knowledge of family medical history is important for its prevention. This disease often skips a generation, but not necessarily. Life-style factors are important in the development and control of this disease. The modern life-style appears to contribute to its prevalence through sedentary life patterns and contemporary diet changes.

Diabetes mellitus is a condition in which there is an inadequate amount of glucose in tissue cells. The reduction of glucose in the cells may be the result of inefficient secretion of insulin by the pancreas or a lowered sensitivity of target cells to insulin. There are two main forms of diabetes mellitus, type I and type II.

Type I or insulin-dependent diabetes mellitus is more common in young people. Persons suffering from type I diabetes require insulin replacement therapy in order to survive.

Type II or non-insulin-dependent diabetes mellitus is most prevalent among older persons and develops more slowly than type I. It occurs principally in persons who are overweight. There may be a genetic predisposition to diabetes. The lower amounts of glucose entering the cells are usually caused by a reduced sensitivity to insulin by the target cells. To offset this resistance, the pancreas generally produces additional amounts of insulin. Thus, persons with type II diabetes may have elevated insulin levels in their blood.

Type II diabetes can be treated through medications, diet modification, and programs of weight control. Exercise is also recommended. Chronic diabetes can cause skin ulcers, glaucoma, cataracts, frequent urination, and loss of weight. Men may experience problems of erectile dysfunction. Diabetes can also interfere with circulation, especially in the extremities. Such circulatory dysfunction can produce gangrene and subsequent amputation of a total limb or partial amputations of toes or feet.

The long-term complications of diabetes mellitus remain a serious health problem. Diabetes mellitus remains a significant public health problem for the elderly. That it is a potent risk factor for the development of premature coronary artery disease, visual impairment, renal failure, neuropathy, and peripheral vascular disease is well-known. Less well-appreciated are the facts that diabetes makes patients admitted to the hospital for any reason at great risk for death than their non-diabetic counterparts of comparable age and sex, and that the risk of death following a myocardial infarction seems to be substantially greater in diabetics than in age- and sex-matched control patients.

Hypothyroidism

The incidence of hypothyroidism increases with age. This condition is difficult to diagnose as symptoms are rather vague and resemble those generally attributed to the general aging process, such as mental confusion. Additional symptoms include fatigue, depression, loss of appetite, weight loss, constipation, and dry skin.

Medical intervention can be quite effective, but, unfortunately, this condition is often inaccurately diagnosed. Such obvious signs such as changes in the skin or nails are often overlooked by health care professionals.

Stress Responses

The physiological changes that persons encounter as they age are not very easily accommodated and can lead to stress. People's ability to respond to stress may alter as they become older. Stressful events for older persons may include the death of a spouse or friends, physical trauma, infection, intense heat or cold, surgical operations, chronic debilitating diseases, family problems, alteration in living arrangements, incontinence, or sensory losses. Several of these stressful events can occur at one time or as clusters over a short period of time. Some of these problems defy solution. Prolonged stress has been linked to the development of Alzheimer's disease. Stressful situations in the lives of the elderly are frequent and often irreversible. This also probably accounts for the high rates of depression found in older adults. It may also provide the roots for suicide in old age.

As far as can be presently determined, the endocrine system in older persons does not materially change with age. Many of the age changes are related to pathological conditions or conditions of lifestyle. Abnormalities of the endocrine system occur long before old age, such as sexual abnormalities or unusual physical characteristics.

Technological Interventions

Older individuals suffer the amputation of toes, feet, or entire limbs. The prognosis for those who refuse such surgical intervention, especially at advanced ages, is extremely poor. Nonetheless, older persons may not consent to amputation. The development of prostheses particularly suited to older amputees is currently being undertaken and new treatment modalities in the rehabilitation of older amputees is being addressed in rehabilitation centers which increasingly serve older clients.

The Immune System

While the immune system is poorly understood, it is well accepted that the immune system plays a significant role in preventing or counteracting the effects of disease. The immune system is crucial to the maintenance of health, particularly with respect to defense against pathogens. Among the numerous physiological defects associated with aging is a generalized decrease in immune function which leads to greater susceptibility to infectious agents, such as bacteria, viruses, fungi, or other foreign substances, as well as to an increase in morbidity and mortality due to infectious disease. This system has received public awareness due to its relationship to the AIDS virus.

The immune system becomes less efficient as people continue to age, and thus they are more susceptible to disease. It is less effective in protecting the body against various bacterial organisms that attack the various systems. It differentiates less effectively between foreign agents that enter the body and the body's own line of defense. Thus, the likelihood of succumbing to disease is increased.

The immune system also includes bone marrow, the thymus gland, the spleen, the lymph nodes, and the tonsils. The role of the tonsils is similar to that of the liver in that it helps in controlling and filtering toxins that enter the body. The movement in the 1930s and 1940s to have children's tonsils removed as a routine health precaution may have compromised the health of these cohorts as they reach the ages of 70 and 80.

Bone marrow located deep in the cavities of bones offers protection against a number of diseases. A diminishment in the amount of bone marrow, along with its alteration in efficiency due to senescence, can compromise the person's health and can lead to death.

White blood cells are part of the body's defense. As people grow older, they become neutralized and are less effective and become destroyed. The result is that older persons are without their protection.

The progressive weakening of the immune system means that the body has fewer and fewer effective defenses to stave off the inroads of disease. The fact that this system is not well understood, neither as it operates in younger or older people, makes it difficult to develop strategies for prevention or intervention. The greater susceptibility of older persons to disease, the pervasive fragility of the older person, leads to its association with the diminished efficiency of the immune system. Understanding the immune system could probably provide significant information on disease prevention and, as a result, ways to extend the life expectancy.

Dysfunctions

The immune system and its interactions are as yet not fully understood. There is insufficient information to determine what specific dysfunctions are related to aging. It appears, however, there is a general decrease in immune sensitivity in older persons. The components of the immune system become less able to recognize the body's own cells in older persons, making them more susceptible to autoimmune responses.

There are a number of diseases that have direct relationship to the malfunctioning of the immune system. AIDS, of course, is one. Older persons are subject to this disease, as well, and this disease presents a problem in some long-term care facilities. The immune system is linked to diseases such as arthritis, cancer, and a variety of infectious diseases. The overall incidence of infectious disease rises in late adulthood. Diseases most prevalent among the elderly are influenza, pneumonia, tuberculosis, meningitis, and urinary tract infections. Cancer increases with age as well, particularly leukemia, lung, prostrate, breast, stomach, and pancreatic cancer.

AIDS is a disease seen in older persons, contracted usually through unsafe sexual practices. There was little effort until recently to educate older persons to the problem of AIDS. Most older women felt that since they were no longer fertile, they did not need to be concerned about contraceptives.

REFERENCES

Chandra, R. (1995). Nutrition and immunity in the elderly: Clinical significance. *Nutrition Review, 53* (4), s80-s85.

Chop, W. C., & Robnett, R. H. (1999). *Gerontology for the Health Professional.* Philadelphia: F.A. Davis.

Lesnoff-Caravaglia, G.(Ed.). (1988). *Handbook of Applied Gerontology.* New York: Human Sciences Press.

Miller, K. (1996). Hormone replacement therapy in the elderly. *Clinical Obstetrics and Gynecology, 39* (4), 912-932.

Oram, J.J. (1997) *Caring for the Fourth Age.* London: Armelle.

Spence, A.D. (1995) *Biology of Human Aging* (2nd ed.). Englewood Cliffs, NJ: Prentice-Hall.

Weksler, M. (1995). Immune senescence: Deficiency or dysregulation. *Nutrition Review, 53* (4), s3-s7.

Wick, G., & Grubeck-Loebenstein, B. (1997). The aging immune system: Primary and secondary alterations of immune reactivity in the elderly. *Experimental Gerontology, 32* (4). 401-413.

Winger, J. & Hornick, T. (1996). Age-associated changes in the endocrine system. *Nursing Clinics of North America, 31* (4), 827-844.

Chapter 11

THE SPECIAL SENSES

Alterations in sensory functioning can affect homeostasis and the quality of life. As persons age, they experience normal sensory changes such as loss of vision, hearing, touch, taste and smell, and, thus, do not absorb as much sensory information from the environment as they did at younger ages. Generally these losses occur at the following ages: vision, age 50; hearing, age 40; touch, age 55; taste, ages 55-59; and smell after age 70. Such changes continue to accelerate with each decade after 65, so that by the late 70s or early 80s, the sensory deterioration may become quite serious.

Special sensory receptors provide a link to the external environment through vision, hearing, equilibrium and balance, taste, and smell. The eyes contain the receptors for vision, the ears those for hearing, equilibrium, and balance. Taste receptors are found in the mouth and throat, and smell in the nose. Touch receptors, as part of the integumentary system, are located throughout the body. Sensory receptors monitor the environment, react to stimuli in the environment, and transmit them to the brain. The stimuli are then registered as tastes, objects, sounds, body position, or smells.

Sensory changes do not begin in everyone at the same age; there are persons who suffer slight or no losses into advanced ages. Sensory changes occur over a period of time, and persons learn to compensate for such losses.

VISION

Adequate vision allows human beings to maintain contact with their environment. Without adequate vision, individuals are isolated from the environment and are almost completely dependent upon others to provide them with mental stimulation. Persons with poor vision often lose interest in the environment, become withdrawn, and depressed. This is particularly true when vision deteriorates late in life, and some older persons are unable to learn new skills such as reading Braille. They are often unable to compensate for their disability.

There is a heavy reliance upon vision to help negotiate the environment. The eye is a very complex organ, and it is composed of a number of elements within the eye that work together to unite it as a unit.

One of these essential elements is the liquid in the eye. This moisture serves several functions. The tear ducts, or lacrimal glands, supply the moisture that washes the eye and keeps it moist, thus preventing the accumulation of foreign particles such as dust or insects. It provides a smooth surface for the muscles of the eye to operate easily, and, through the blinking of the eye, the fluid is spread across the eye.

The drying of this liquid in the eye is an age-related problem that can cause pain and irritation. To offset the malfunctioning of the lacrimal glands, substitute tears and liquids to provide moisture and to cleanse the eye are frequently prescribed. The drying of the eye can also result from various disease states, such as fevers.

There are a number of muscles in the eye. They are important to the internal functioning of the eye, and also for the opening and closing of the eyelids. The diminishment of muscle strength in the eye leads to conditions which can impair vision. Some muscle changes are related to the presence of disease, but some are due to senescence. There is a loss of fat and elastic tissue from around the eyes and a thinning of the skin in the eyelids. This causes the formation of wrinkles at the corners of the eyes. The loss of elasticity also produces many loose folds of skin that form pouches under the eyes. Objects may be perceived less rapidly. The general movement of the eye can be slowed; this is also true of the raising and lowering of eyelids. For some older people the eyelid does not close completely, and this can result in sleep disturbances and dry eyes.

The cornea of the eye becomes less of a sphere and becomes a little flatter in old age. There is a yellowing of the lens as well, and not as much light reaches the retina. The pupil does not dilate as openly or fully; approximately one third of the light does not reach photoreceptors in the back of the eye, resulting in decreased input to the brain.

This accounts for older person's requiring more light than do younger persons to read or to carry out activities effectively.

The yellowing of the lens also affects color perception of such hues as blues and greens. Such changes can also lead to faulty color perception, such as the mismatching of colors in clothing, and is potentially embarrassing.

Failure of vision with age results from changes in the eye itself—the surrounding muscles and the central nervous system. Three major changes in the eye begin to occur in the mid-50s. The lens of the eye becomes increasingly rigid and opaque and gradually yellows. The surrounding eye muscles begin to weaken and to become more lax. As a result of these physical changes, several problems occur—a decrease in visual acuity, or the ability to see objects clearly, a decrease in the ability to focus on objects at different distances, a decrease in the ability to discern certain color intensities and a decrease in the ability to judge distances.

Visual acuity reflects how clearly objects can be seen. In order to have 20/20, or normal vision, a person must stand 20 feet from an eye chart and be able to distinguish figures of a particular size. Visual acuity is relatively undeveloped in young children, and optimal acuity is achieved in young adulthood. This explains why children require large type in order to read more easily. From the mid-20s to approximately age 50, there is a slight decline in visual acuity, and, from that age onwards, the decline is accelerated. It is not uncommon to have an 80 percent loss of visual acuity by the age of 85.

Another visual change is that of accommodation or the ability of the eye to focus on the detail of objects at varying distances. One example where loss of accommodation might have an effect is while driving through the busy center of a city where one must focus on different objects at different distances, such as signs, pedestrians, automobiles, and traffic lights. With aging, the accommodation or the ability to shift or quickly change focus becomes slightly delayed.

Another aspect of accommodation is the ability to focus on objects that are close at hand. Due to age related changes, some older people will be able to read more clearly the fine print in newspapers when held at some distance compensating for a decline in visual accommodation.

Another visual problem relates to the amount of light or illumination needed to enable an older person to see effectively. As persons age they require increased amounts of light. Generally, persons age 80 require approximately three times more light to read a book than that needed by persons in their teens. Compounding this problem is the fact that the elderly experience an exaggerated amount of glare from an intense light source. Thus merely increasing the amount of light by using a stronger light bulb serves to further decrease the older person's ability to see. To minimize the extreme glare and to make the environment more functional, evenly distributed or balanced light sources are an important consideration.

Related to the problem of light levels, is the fact that an older person has difficulty seeing clearly in the dark or in dimly lit areas. In addition, sight recovery is delayed when moving from a light environment to a dark environment or vice versa. This is known as dark adaptation. In long-term care settings, residents moving from their darkened rooms into a brighter hallway can experience falls due to diminished ability to adapt to differing light levels. The glare from floors or walls also compromises their adaptation, as well as their inability to see the handrail.

A clouding or yellowing of the lens occurs resulting in another vision problem in the inability to discern color intensities clearly. This occurs primarily when colors are closely related particularly in the deep blue, green and violet end of the color spectrum. Colors tend to fade and blend. Red, yellow, and orange are generally more easily seen. This loss in the ability to see certain color intensities clearly decreases the older person's depth perception which is the ability to judge distances. Judging the difference between steps may be difficult when the landing, stairs, and walls are of the same color intensity.

Decreased visual acuity or the ability to see objects clearly, decreased ability to focus on objects at different distances, decreased ability to function in lower light levels and to discern certain color intensities and to judge distances are all normal age-related visual losses.

These gradual losses generally have an overall negative impact on the functional vision of the older person. This occurs some time in the late 70s. When this happens, the person's visual perception is distorted, and the ability to visually select certain critical information from a new environment is severely affected. This may affect the person's independent functioning or the desire to seek out new social situations. Some people, however, maintain nearly normal sight well into old age.

Dysfunctions

Presbyopia

Presbyopia or farsightedness is probably the most common age-related dysfunction of the eye. The effects of presbyopia are usually noted at approximately age 40. Its occurrence is so universal that it is regarded as a normal senescent change. Presbyopia is not a disease, but a degenerative change that occurs in the aging eye.

In this condition, there is a gradual loss of lens elasticity. In addition, there is a flattening of the shape of the lens and an increase in density. Consequently, the lens has a diminished ability to change shape and to bend the light rays for viewing near objects. The accommodation for near vision is either absent or greatly reduced. Such changes generally occur by the age of 55.

Because of presbyopia, most people need reading glasses or bifocals by the time they are in their 50s. There are persons, however, who do not experience this change in vision and enjoy normal eyesight into advanced old age. Instances of persons in their 80s or 90s performing activities such as sewing or reading without the benefit of visual aids have been documented.

Blindness

The incidence of blindness increases with age due to the number of diseases that can precipitate this condition. The most common causes of blindness in old age are diabetic retinopathy, glaucoma, and cataracts.

Glaucoma

The most serious eye disease in old age is glaucoma; its cause is an elevated pressure within the eye. If untreated, glaucoma can cause blindness. It is reported to be the second leading cause of blindness in the United States.

Although it is not totally clear why glaucoma develops, eye disease or injury are common causes. Persons can also inherit a predisposition to the condition. Usually glaucoma is a disease of slow onset and progression. Unfortunately, it develops at such a slow rate that the eye may be seriously damaged before the person seeks medical assistance.

Symptoms include blurred vision, the experience of pain, and watering of the eye. Additional symptoms may include severe headache, dizziness, and nausea. A gradual loss of peripheral vision, usually affecting both eyes simultaneously, is usually the first sign. The visual field may eventually become so restricted that persons only see objects that are in their direct line of vision. They are left with what is known as tunnel vision. Untreated, the condition gradually worsens, and total blindness is the result.

There is no cure for glaucoma. The pressure within the eye can be relieved through medication, eye drops, or surgery. Marijuana is frequently prescribed as a treatment for glaucoma.

Diabetic Retinopathy

People who suffer from diabetes can also experience diabetic retinopathy. Diabetes is frequently first diagnosed by an optometrist during a routine eye examination. Diabetic retinopathy can result in blindness.

Symptoms include clouding of vision and seeing spots or dots of light before the eyes. The condition develops very gradually and can cover a period of years. Eventually, vision is seriously affected, and the end result is blindness.

A predisposition to diabetes mellitus can be inherited, and it appears that this condition skips generations. If it appears in grandparents, children are less likely to inherit the condition, but it may well appear in grandchildren. This disease does not strictly follow this pattern, but it is sufficiently common that parents should monitor their children's health closely and include periodic eye examinations if the disease is part of the family medical history.

Cataracts

Cataracts are the most common disability of the aged eye. An increase in the number of elderly people is accompanied by a greater incidence of this disorder. Cataracts seem to be a consequence of aging; their incidence increases progressively after age 50 and approaches 95 percent of the population 85 years or older. In the United States, cataracts account for more than half of the hospitalizations caused by eye disorders, and the cataract operation is the single most common surgical procedure done in this country. The crystalline lens of a normal eye sometimes becomes opaque, often as a consequence of aging. This condition is termed a cataract. Once a cataract has been removed, a lens substitute must be used to restore vision. The substitute may be a lens placed in front of the eye (spectacles), on the surface of the eye (contact lens), or inside the eyes (intraocular lens). For many persons, intraocular lenses may be more effective than the other lenses, but may also involve greater risks. Even though cataract surgery is a rather simple procedure and has a high success rate, there continue to be cases of blindness due to cataracts.

Although cataracts are fairly common, they were once considered a serious condition that called for hospitalization. Cataracts can now be easily and successfully treated in ambulatory care centers.

Age-Related Macular Degeneration

Age-related macular degeneration is the leading cause of legal blindness among older adults, especially women. There are also indications that it may be genetic. It is a disease in which the eye's macula, a remarkably sensitive structure in the middle of the retina, gradually loses its ability to distinguish shapes and colors. While not a fatal disorder, it can be extremely debilitating. Although the macula (named after the Latin word for spot) is no wider than a pencil, it is a hundred times more sensitive to small-scale features than the rest of the retina. Without a healthy macula, people cannot read a newspaper, recognize a friend, thread a needle, watch TV, safely negotiate stairs, or see much of anything at all.

Until now, physicians have been able to offer only palliative care to patients with macular degeneration: more powerful eyeglasses; visual aids, such as machines that enlarge print; and, for a minority of cases—those that involve the invasive growth of blood vessels—laser therapy that sometimes slows down the disease, at least for a time.

Macular degeneration is devastating because it kills off a small but critical patch of light-sensing cells that line the retina like the film in a camera. Known as rods and cones because of their telltale shapes, these cells record visual images as patterns of illumination and shadow, and relay that information, as electrical impulses, through the optic nerve to the brain. It is not that people with macular degeneration become completely blind; peripheral vision, which is handled by other areas of the retina, remains unaffected by the disease. However, as damage to the macula builds up—probably a consequence of chemical damage that accumulates over a lifetime—central vision fades, making it difficult to distinguish fine detail of the objects viewed. The external world dissolves into an indistinct blur.

The disease process does not attack the macula's light-sensing cells directly. It starts in the layer of tissue that lies just below them. The cells that constitute this tissue are known as retinal pigment epithelium (RPE) cells. These cells provide the light-sensing cells with nourishment and dispose of their wastes. RPE cells, however, cannot replace themselves through cell division. Thus, when the RPE cells begin to sicken and die, so do the cells they support.

Leading ophthalmologists have recently begun exploring the possibility of replacing the dysfunctional RPE cells with healthy fetal cells. Cells from the retina of an aborted fetus are surgically transplanted into impaired eyes. The transplanted cells proliferate, forming minute projections that stretch toward the diseased macula. Fetal RPE cells can divide and thus increase in number.

Unfortunately, most cases of age-related macular degeneration do not respond to medical or surgical treatment. The use of magnifying devices—either hand-held or incorporated into eyeglass lenses—has proved beneficial in overcoming some of the loss of visual acuity. Because only the macular region of the retina is affected, this condition does not cause the person to become completely blind.

Research suggests that it is familial or genetic and that environmental factors, with the passage of time, make the disease one that is evident in old age. Diabetes mellitus, hypertension, and high cholesterol also affect this region of the eye. The development of macular degeneration may be related to those conditions in some persons.

Accidents

Many alterations in vision are the result of accidents. Older individuals are particularly susceptible to accidents, and many such injuries affect the eyes. The exercise of caution and employing safety measures can significantly reduce the eye injuries and preserve vision in old age. Accidents in the home are the prime causes of injury. Rugs that are not skid-proof, dimly lit stairways, and unsafe bathrooms are common causes of falls. Economic measures conducted by older people such as not using electricity to provide sufficient light can lead to fatal injuries. Environmental factors frequently produce more problems in terms of health care than do the actual physical changes brought on by senescence.

Vision and Technology

Many people maintain their vision into advanced old age. The presence of new interventions in terms of surgical procedures (laser surgery), new types of glasses, contact lenses, industrial safety, and better understanding of preventive measures have all led to improved vision in old age. The maintenance of general good health, particularly the cardiovascular system, improves the conditions and functioning of the visual apparatus in old age.

One of the most innovative devices is the development of the robot-dog that takes the place of the guide dog. In appearance it resembles a large vacuum cleaner with a long handle. The long handle keeps the user in contact with the mechanism as it moves through space avoiding obstacles. Derived from a model used in industry, this mechanism can be equipped with lights for nighttime use, sound elements, and attachments to suit individual needs.

HEARING

Impaired hearing is common among older individuals. Some loss is due to age-related physiological change in the auditory system, and some is due to disease and superimposed environmental insults. There is great variability in the decline of hearing. The ear contains receptors that transform sound waves into nerve impulses that are interpreted as sounds by the brain, as well as receptors providing information concerning balance and equilibrium.

The ear is made up of three sections: the external, the middle and the inner ear. The external ear collects the sound waves that are then interpreted by the brain, the middle ear contains the ear drum, the inner ear contains the temporal bone which is frequently the site for ear implants to offset hearing problems. Sounds are the result of vibrations that travel over the fluid that is present in the ear.

The accumulation of excessive earwax can affect the hearing of an older person. Approximately one-third of the instances of hearing losses in the low-frequency tones in older persons is due to the buildup of earwax.

It is dangerous for persons to attempt to remove the wax as there is the potential for puncturing the ear drum. Wax accumulation can be safely removed by a physician, and hearing is restored.

Most changes in the outer ear do not affect hearing. This is also the case with respect to the middle-ear structures. The initiation of hearing loss usually occurs by the age of 40. It is due primarily to changes within the structures of the inner ear.

The vestibulocochlear nerve is made up of two sections. The cochlear section is related to hearing. The vestibular section is connected to balance and equilibrium. After the age of 45, there are alterations, not only in hearing, but in those areas which affect balance and equilibrium, as well. Problems of balance and equilibrium are particularly evident after the age of 70.

Hearing loss is gradual and occurs at about middle age, and is more common among males than females. It is not clear why men experience hearing loss earlier, but it could be due to environmental factors such as industrial noise or listening to certain forms of music.

Dysfunctions

Hearing loss is a major problem for the elderly. National surveys show that hearing impairment is the third most prevalent chronic condition among the non-institutionalized elderly, exceeded only by arthritis and hypertensive disease.

Hearing impaired individuals include both those who are deaf and those who are hard of hearing. Hard of hearing refers to a degree of hearing impairment that interferes with comprehension of speech, although partial auditory function remains. Deaf refers to a degree of impairment that renders hearing non-functional for the ordinary purposes of life. Even the partial loss of hearing that is often associated with aging can limit independence and negatively affect quality of life for the elderly. Hearing loss restricts the individual's ability to interact with others and to give, receive, and interpret information. Sound is important for self-protection and identification of hazards in the environment. Ultimately, hearing loss can affect mental and physical health, decreasing the ability of some individuals to function independently and increasing the need for formal and informal long-term care services. Hearing impairment rises sharply with age.

Types of hearing impairment include conductive, sensorineural, mixed, and central hearing impairments. These types are based on the site of structural damage or blockage. Conductive hearing impairment involves the outer and/or middle ear. Sensorineural impairment involves damage to the inner ear, the cochlea, and/or fibers of the eighth cranial nerve. A mixed hearing impairment is one that comprises both conductive and sensorineural components. A central processing disorder is a hearing impairment that influences the understanding of spoken language; the elderly person may hear the words but be unable to make sense of them as a result of disorders of the auditory pathways in the brain.

Another problem often seen in older persons with hearing loss is recruitment, an inability to tolerate loud sounds. This condition can interfere with satisfactory use of a hearing aid.

Tinnitus

Tinnitus is the perception of constant background noise generated in the ears or head. It can be present in one or both ears. This is commonly referred to as ringing of the ears, but the sound may also be described as buzzing, whirring, humming, or other annoying sound that seems, once it is initiated, never leaves.

Although the noise is generated somewhere within the auditory system, it is not clear what mechanisms are involved. Other causes of tinnitus may be infection of the middle ear structures, meningitis, high blood pressure, or cardiovascular diseases. There is some suggestion that persons who use the telephone extensively are prone to developing tinnitus.

Many conditions that alter the central nervous system can cause tinnitus, but the single most common cause is degeneration of cochlear or auditory nerve function. The prevalence of tinnitus increases with age. It is usually accompanied by some degree of hearing loss.

Tinnitus seems to be more common in women. Many people become irritable and impatient more easily because they have to deal with this inner confusion, while at the same time dealing with the problems of daily life. A "sour" look or one of constant irritation can become the typical facial expression of a person suffering from tinnitus.

The development of implants which produce the sound similar to the crackling of frying bacon help to offset the constant noise produced by tinnitus. At bedtime some persons listen to radio stations that produce static in order to fall asleep. The static seems to counteract the sound in the ears. There is no known cure for tinnitus due to nerve degeneration. Tinnitus may become quite severe; there are anecdotal reports of suicide because of this condition.

Deafness

Although large numbers of older persons experience hearing impairment, deafness, or the total loss of hearing, is rare. As persons advance in age, deafness becomes more common. There are two forms of deafness: conductive deafness and nerve deafness.

Conductive deafness results when transmission of sound waves is hindered or blocked. For this condition, hearing aids that are helpful are those that transmit sound waves to the inner ear through the bone of the skull.

Nerve deafness is the loss of hearing from disorders that affect the receptor cells of the spiral organ, the neurons of the vestibulocochlear nerve, or nerve pathways within the central nervous system. In these cases, regular hearing aids are of little avail. Instead cochlear implants can be used. Cochlear implants are extremely useful to counteract nerve deafness, but the sounds do not equate with normal hearing.

Dizziness and Vertigo

The level of liquid in the ear can be paralleled to a carpenter's level. The bubble in the center of the level has to remain constant for there to be a level reading. This lack of a level reading in the ear, causes dysfunctions such as dizziness and vertigo. Dizziness is usually described as an unsteadiness or lack of spatial relationship. In vertigo, the experience is one in which either the world is spinning around the person, or the person is spinning about in space.

Older persons are more likely to experience dizziness or vertigo, and it is a common complaint. These conditions can be caused by an inflammation within the inner ear which is related to balance and equilibrium or of an inflammation of the nerve fibers of the vestibulo-cochlear nerve. Vertigo is usually a symptom of inner ear disease.

Benign vertigo which does not appear to be linked to pathology is not well understood. There is some indication that persons who suffer this condition should not look upward for long periods of time or to crook the neck backwards. The theory (basilar artery insufficiency) is that blockage of arteries carrying oxygen to the cerebellum causes the experience of vertigo. The use of aspirin on a daily basis seems to alleviate symptoms for some individuals.

Problems of balance can be linked to various disease states such as diabetes. Diabetics frequently suffer dizziness and walk listing to one side. They may go into a coma and fall onto the sidewalk or in the street, and be mistaken for being under the influence of alcohol.

Presbycusis

With aging comes a gradual, progressive hearing loss which is known as presbycusis ("old hearing"), a sensorineural loss resulting from changes in the inner ear. It occurs in both ears, but the rate of loss may be different in each ear. Some researchers believe that presbycusis is associated with normal aging, while others believe it results primarily from disease conditions. Not all elderly individuals have presbycusis, and some people in their 90s retain acute hearing.

Although, presbycusis is a progressive loss of hearing, the symptoms are not readily apparent until the person is over age 65. The loss is complicated by other factors such as illnesses, substance abuse, and noise. Men are affected more than women, and urban dwellers suffer greater losses than those living in rural areas. Long-term exposure to environmental noise may contribute significantly to the development of presbycusis. This may be truer of men because of the industrial settings in which many men work. The degree of loss is more severe for high-frequency sounds than for low-frequency sounds. The selective loss of high-frequency hearing makes it difficult for older persons to hear consonants. Such changes also cause speech to sound muffled. Some older persons compensate for this loss by lip-reading. Also, hearing conversations in a crowded room can pose difficulties for older persons because of their additionally diminished ability to localize sound and to mask sounds that are considered less important.

In the average person over age 65, the effects of presbycusis can be summarized as having two general tendencies: an inability to hear higher frequencies and a reduced ability to hear sound in general. To an older person speech may sound garbled and difficult to understand, or muffled. Parts of words become unintelligible. This apparently occurs as word sounds go above the 2000 cycle frequency and are thus filtered out or not heard. Merely speaking louder to an aged individual may not make speech easier for them to understand because high frequency sounds continue to be filtered out. For example, background noise such as noises from appliances, television or busy public places are low frequency noises, and, as such, interfere further with the older person's ability to hear normal conversation.

Along with the presence of severe loss due to presbycusis, an older person may have the additional difficulty of understanding speech. The person may be mistakenly labelled as mentally impaired or as suffering from dementia, when the person actually only has presbycusis.

There are many theories and disagreements as to what actually causes presbycusis. Since presbycusis almost universally affects the hearing of the elderly, the increases in life expectancy indicate that presbycusis will become a common problem for future older populations. Such widespread hearing loss can have a major effect on how people will behave in the future in both social and physical environments.

Hearing Impairment

Poor vision in old age may interfere with lip-reading techniques the individual, who has been deaf from childhood, has used successfully throughout life. The elderly who become hearing impaired late in life present different problems because they must acquire an entirely new and complex system of communication in order to maintain social interaction.

Hearing impairment causes social and psychological difficulties by interfering with the individual's ability to communicate with family and friends. This can lead to withdrawal, social isolation, and depression. Loss of hearing interferes with the elderly person's ability to compensate for other losses that can occur with aging, such as loss of relationships due to the death of a spouse, siblings, and friends, loss of a familiar home or community, and worsening health and mobility. Lack of easy communication means decreased access to new people, new activities, and new services.

Hearing impairment limits access to information that is normally available through personal communication, telephone, radio, and television. For elderly individuals who have both hearing and visual impairments, access to information is often severely limited, and some research indicates that restricted access to information can contribute to the progressive development of confusion. There is also, unfortunately, the widespread assumption that older persons who are hearing impaired are also confused.

Hearing impairment is often not seen as important by the elderly, their families, and health care providers. Denial of hearing impairment and failure to recognize its impact on independent functioning are clear obstacles to effective treatment. Hearing impairment is not visible, and invisibility facilitates denial.

Treatment of Hearing Impairment

Treatment of hearing impairment includes methods to either prevent hearing impairment or to reduce its severity or to improve the individual's communicative competence through amplification or other electronic and mechanical devices. In addition, public facilities can be adapted to accommodate the special needs of hearing impaired persons. People can also be educated on how to manage their hearing problems through the provision of information about devices and other compensatory strategies to reduce communication handicaps.

Prevention

Too little is known about the causes of hearing loss associated with aging to allow effective preventive measures. Some hearing impairments in older people result from preventable problems that began earlier in life, such as untreated infections and exposure to noise. Some drugs damage auditory mechanisms. Aspirin can be ototoxic, though probably only in the high dosage levels sometimes used in the treatment of arthritis. Aspirin-induced hearing loss is usually reversible if it is recognized early and dosage is reduced.

The likelihood of curing hearing impairments in the elderly with available medical or surgical treatment is limited because they are almost always sensorineural losses, most of which are currently not treatable.

Environmental Factors Affecting Visual and Hearing Loss

Since changes in vision and hearing occur gradually, and within the context of the normal aging process, older persons are able to adjust to such changes with some success. There are, however, environmental factors which influence the ability of the older person to accomplish the activities of everyday life. Such environmental factors may be positive or negative.

Normal age-related hearing and vision losses can have a dramatic effect on the older person's ability to function even in a familiar physical and social environment. Such gradual sensory changes have a profound effect on the daily life of the elderly.

For some, clothing selection may be a problem since colors, particularly blues and greens, tend to fade and blend. The loss of the ability to focus clearly can create problems in the use of appliances. Temperature settings on irons or microwaves, for example, can be difficult to read.

Hearing loss appears to have a more serious affect on the social participation of older persons. They feel separated from the world due to the loss of hearing, and have a tendency to withdraw. They are more fearful of the environment because warning signs for the deaf are not as prevalent to announce dangers, caution, or safety features. The absolute silence that can surround the person can be difficult to reconcile.

Older persons suffering vision loss, seem to maintain a higher level of social participation than do those who experience hearing losses. Voices of loved ones can be heard, nuances of speech are enjoyed, and the comfort level in terms of the ability to deal with the environment seems to be higher with the visually impaired.

Prevention and Intervention

Although a certain amount of hearing loss might be inevitable and attributed to the aging process, there are many approaches to intervention that can be noted. Medical and surgical advances report impact on the elimination of hearing loss, or the reduction of the extent of loss. Examples are the miracle drugs' effects upon mastoid infections and the perfection of microsurgery in the treatment of otosclerosis. Legal intervention, such as the Occupational Safety and Health Administration (OSHA) regulations on reasonable constraints on noise in the workplace, represents an attempt to meet the problem at its source in order to prevent damage. The hearing-aid industry places great importance on its research-and-development programs in the attempt to produce hearing aids that give greater fidelity to the sound and that extend the range of the frequency response. Knowing the wishes of the consumers, the industry attempts to make such improvements while attending to cosmetic factors. This is a large area for potential growth in terms of intervention, since it is known that only a small percentage of those who could benefit from amplification are actual users of hearing aids. Hearing aids are amplification devices designed to compensate for partial hearing loss.

Continued research in the area of cochlear implants can lead to improvements for the profoundly hard-of-hearing population. Intervention also is found in the increase in the availability of assistive listening devices other than hearing aids. Such intervention includes the FM broadcasting by a teacher or minister in a classroom or a church that is transmitted to a receiving mechanism worn by the hard-of-hearing listener. Many theaters now have special infrared amplification systems in which the actors' voices are picked up at the stage level and broadcast into the auditorium, where the sound can be received by a special listening device worn by the person who is hard-of-hearing. These, and other assistive listening devices, are designed to overcome problems that are present in certain communication situations where a conventional hearing aid does not prove to be adequate to the task.

TASTE

Loss of taste is a common complaint among older persons. This can be caused by atrophy of the taste buds which comes with age, or by lesions of the facial nerve and the brain.

Taste is a chemical sense that is taken for granted, and its importance is often underestimated. Changes in taste perception can affect the quality and quantity of the foods that people consume. Receptors for taste or taste buds are found on the tongue, the inside of the cheeks, in the throat, and on the roof of the mouth.

Diseases in these areas, such as cancers, can result in taste alterations. Oral health is important in preserving the sense of taste. Lifestyle factors such as abuse of alcohol, other drugs (including medications), and tobacco can all change taste perception. The sense of taste accounts for only four of the sensations that many people call flavors; all other flavors are due to the sense of smell. There are four primary taste sensations: salty, sour, sweet, and bitter. Aging seems to cause slight decreases only in the ability to detect salty and bitter substances. The amount of change is highly variable among individuals, and the ability to detect salt declines the most. The degree of taste impairment seems to vary from taste to taste, being less pronounced for sweet and most profound for salt.

Losses in taste can have serious consequences for older persons as the maintenance of proper nutritional levels is vital to their physical and mental well-being. Older persons frequently state that food lacks flavor. Disinterest in eating can also reflect loneliness, grief, or the onset of an illness.

Although there is a general decrease in taste perception, older persons retain the ability to taste certain substances and not others. Such taste alterations may be due to a decline in the number of taste buds. Diminished taste perception can also be linked to changes in the processing of taste sensations in the central nervous system.

Other contributing factors to the reduction of the sensation of taste in older persons are decreases in the amount of saliva in the oral cavity and changes in the surface texture of the tongue. Medication can alter the taste of food. Life-style factors such as abuse of alcohol or years of addiction to cigarette smoking can contribute to the decrease.

Taste perception can be enhanced through oral sprays that provide moisture to the mouth. They also help in the dissolving of food. The addition of various herbs to food preparations can make food more palatable to older persons.

SMELL

A decline of the sense of smell (hyposmia) in older persons can carry serious consequences. Much like taste, there are variations in the ability to smell particular odors. The ability to distinguish individual odors in a mixture appears to be gradually lost as a person ages. Such losses in the sense of smell seem to have a greater effect upon men than women.

Aging causes decreases in the number of sensory neurons for smell. These neurons are called olfactory neurons and are located in the upper portion of the nasal cavities. Aging also causes deterioration of the pathways that carry olfactory impulses through the brain. All these changes cause a decline in the ability to detect and identify aromas. The degree of change is highly variable among individuals.

Since much of what is commonly referred to as flavor is actually aroma, age changes in the sense of smell reduce the pleasure derived from eating and can contribute to malnutrition. The sense of smell is of particular importance in older persons because of its close relationship with the sense of taste. For a person to enjoy food and to eat a balanced diet, the food must have an inviting taste. In order for food to have a satisfying taste, it must also appeal to the sense of smell. The sense of smell helps whet the appetite, and thus creates a linkage between the senses of taste and smell.

Olfactory sensory cells, like taste receptors, are replaced by new cells as they die. Although poorly understood and insufficiently researched, the sense of smell begins to alter in middle age and progressively declines as persons age.

Persons with a long history of cigarette smoking are more prone to alterations in smell perception. Reduced olfaction also means a reduced ability to detect harmful aromas such as toxic fumes and dangerous gases.

The protective measures provided by the sense of smell are considerable. The diminishment or loss of this sense in old age is a major detriment to independent functioning. Environmental cues such as the presence of gas or burning substances can be overlooked. A kitchen range can function improperly, and the escaping gas not noticed. Food that is spoiled or harmful can be ingested by the person with an inadequate sense of taste or smell.

Sanitation measures may not be followed as rigorously as the sense of smell is diminished. Personal bathing may not be as frequent. The performance of daily tasks such as garbage removal may lapse. The living environment may not be aired and may become odorous and unhealthy. Finally, a declining ability to notice offensive odors can lead to socially embarrassing situations.

TOUCH

The sense of touch has not been given serious consideration with respect to its importance in understanding the environment. Touch receptors and pressure receptors in the skin decrease in number and become structurally distorted as persons age.

Such changes can lead to a decreased ability to notice that something is touching the person or the ability to recognize an object by touch. Decreases in the ability to detect, locate, and identify objects touching or pressing on the skin result in decreases in the ability to respond to those objects and can lead to accidents. As a consequence, harmful objects may be encountered more frequently, more severely, and for longer periods. Reduced sensation may also mean reduced pleasure from favorable physical contact, and this can have psychological and social consequences.

Although nerve endings in the skin are not greatly affected anatomically with age, some changes in nerve tissue do occur. Changes as persons age seem to reflect a diminished sensitivity to pressure and light touch or surface contexts such as textures and surface differences. Pain perception and pain reaction thresholds are somewhat reduced. Reactions to hot or cold objects appear to be delayed, resulting in unintentional injuries such as burns. In general, the ability to sense danger tactilely and to respond accordingly is reduced. Reductions in sensation from the skin seem to result from a weakening in the conduction of impulses to the cortical nervous system.

Sensory Loss and Negative Stereotyping

Sensory loss can be experienced over an extended period of time, and its onset is gradual. It is, however, most apparent in older persons. There is a general cultural impatience with persons who do not function at expected levels. When persons suffer from hearing loss, for example, they are often thought to be mentally impaired.

Older persons who suffer from the loss of several senses at one time, also experience negative attitudes. Since attitudes find their reflection in behaviors, older persons often do not fare well because of these disabilities. Because of hearing or vision losses, they are at times viewed not as persons, but as objects within the environment. Such objectivity, particularly on the part of health and social service providers, can further compromise the physical and mental health of older persons.

Social and psychological factors that discourage use of a hearing aid include reluctance to call attention to the hearing impairment and disappointment with the quality of sound provided by the hearing aid. Individuals who once had normal hearing often expect that a hearing aid will return their hearing to normal, and the disappointment they experience in trying to adjust to a hearing aid can create significant acceptance problems.

Because a number of older persons experience difficulty in adjusting to the use of hearing aids, this is often viewed as a rejection of or an inability to adjust to something new. In reality, many older persons do not use their hearing aids simply because the aids are inappropriate for their hearing impairments.

Telecommunications Systems

One of the most common and frequent problems for hearing impaired older individuals is the inability to use the telephone. This problem is compounded for those who experience visual as well as hearing losses. For older persons, particularly for the great numbers who live alone, the telephone is a link to the outside world; inability to use the telephone can compromise safety and interfere with independent functioning.

Hearing over the telephone is difficult even for those with mild hearing loss because telephone signal transmission omit very low- and high frequency sounds that are important for understanding speech.

Line noises and other sound distortions also interfere with the quality of sound transmission.

Devices to assist hearing impaired individuals to use the telephone include amplifiers that can be built into the telephone handset or attached to the side of the telephone. Telecoils can also be built into hearing aids to pick up electronic signals directly from the telephone receiver, bypassing the hearing aid microphone.

The development of effective computerized speech recognition systems could greatly simplify telephone use for the hearing impaired. These systems convert spoken words into printed output that is then displayed on a screen attached to the telephone. Currently available speech recognition systems still have major limitations.

Signaling and Alarm Systems

Signaling and alarm systems that convert sound to visual or tactile signals are important for the safety and independence of hearing impaired persons. Flashing lights and vibrating devices that signal the ringing of a fire alarm, smoke alarm, telephone, doorbell, or alarm clock substitute for sounds the person cannot hear. Tactile paging devices use radio signals to generate vibrations in a portable receiver carried by the hearing impaired individual.

Since older persons are seldom part of the informal deaf community, they are unaware of the availability of such devices. They usually do not receive comprehensive aural rehabilitation services, and, as a result, are not informed about available devices from hearing specialists.

Environmental Design

Building design characteristics affect the behavior of sound and the relative ease or difficulty of hearing. For example, hard-surfaced walls and floor reflect sound, creating reverberations that interfere with hearing, while sound-absorbent wall covering materials decrease reverberations.

While much is known about design characteristics that affect hearing, this information is seldom applied in buildings used by the elderly. Reduction of reverberations and background noise in these facilities could considerably ameliorate some of the problems of those with hearing loss.

Service Providers

Hearing services for the elderly are provided primarily by physicians, audiologists, and hearing aid dealers. Physician evaluation is important to identify impairments that are medically treatable, but physicians usually receive little training in the management of hearing impairments and alternative approaches to compensate for hearing loss.

Audiologists are non-medical specialists trained in the identification and evaluation of hearing impairment and rehabilitation of individuals with hearing deficits. Many older individuals enter the service delivery system through a hearing aid dealer. When they are fitted with hearing aids without consulting an audiologist, they run the risk of purchasing an aid that may be totally inappropriate.

The prevalence of hearing loss in older persons far exceeds that of most chronic diseases and disabilities of later life, but the magnitude of this problem has not been reflected in the amount of research that has been conducted in pathology, prevention, treatment, and rehabilitation. Hearing impairment in old age is often mild or moderate; it is often progressive. Hearing impairment in the elderly often coexists with other health problems that complicate treatment and limit the effectiveness of available assistive devices.

Denial of hearing impairment on the part of the older person is a continuing obstacle to treatment. The most effective method of treatment available at present is the use of devices and techniques that compensate for hearing loss. An assortment of signaling devices exist to provide either tactile or visual cues to phone rings, doorbells, clock alarms, smoke alarms, door knocks, or cries of an infant. Strobe-type fire alarms, flashing phone ringers, and doorbell flashers are inexpensive and have been available for some time. There are, however, few distributors for many such devices, and too few of those who could possibly benefit know about what the devices do and how one acquires them. Marketing typically concentrates on advertisement through specialized journals, which are unfamiliar to the average hearing-disabled older person.

Vision

Problems posed by blindness and by low vision have prompted the development of new technology. One example is the Kurzweil Reading Machine; it can read aloud a book or magazine. Some people can learn to read text via Optacon (Telesensory Systems, Inc.), which converts print to a vibrating tactile pattern on the fingertip. A long cane still is relatively inexpensive, and with proper training, it affords a good deal of independent mobility. Talking books, radio, and the new flood of literature recorded on standard audiocassettes (designed for general consumption) offer some solutions to loss of reading ability.

Low vision may be functionally defined as loss of visual acuity or visual field severe enough to prevent performance of a desired task. Most of the severely vision-impaired older population have residual vision that may be optimized by comprehensive low-vision services. Such services are typically provided through clinics specializing in low vision.

Tactile Impairment and Technology

There are a few technologies that may be employed to the benefit of those who are "touch-blind." Special gloves that indicate excessive cumulative pressure by color change generated when dye-containing microcapsules rupture may be worn during repetitive tasks. A few simple experimental systems, designed for measuring cumulative pressures at points in the sole, provide audible alerts once a certain critical threshold is passed. Attempts to design systems that provide a form of artificial skin sensation have been unsuccessful to date. Sensory substitution (or, rather, sensory transfer) technology could allow development of an unobtrusive appliance, built into footwear or glove, that transmits relevant haptic information electrically to transducers placed on areas of sensitive skin.

The impact of common age-related changes in touch sensibility is related to decline in sensory thresholds. Decreased sensitivity and position sense in aging are thought to be related to changes in the skin itself, receptors within the skin, and changes in the nervous system. Decreased tactile sensitivity in blind diabetics has been cited as a barrier to the use of Braille and other tactile vision aids. Despite diminished sensibility at the fingertips, blind adults can be taught enough Braille to assist in activities of daily living.

Polymodal Sensory Disorder

The effects of combined impairments in more than one sensory system in the older adult have been understudied. Older diabetics have been known to experience dizziness or lightheadedness when walking. Spatial disorientation can result from multisensory loss and vestibular-visual mismatch through improper eyewear.

Multiple sensory losses may contribute to confusional states among the hospitalized elderly. Such problems often result in medical intervention (e.g., administration of major tranquilizers) when correction of underlying impairments, adjustment of environment, or personal one-one-one supervision might be safer and more effective interventions.

The effects of chronic sensory deprivation in the frail elderly are unknown. Sensory deprivation and social isolation may reinforce each other and sometimes contribute to both general disorientation and decline in cognitive function. It is possible that intellectual deterioration may be at least partially reversible by facilitating sensory information and socially reengaging people.

Future Technological Developments

The sense of touch begins to assume major importance when other sensory channels are less efficient. Regardless of how advanced cochlear prostheses become, it remains likely that there will always be a population for whom a tactile hearing substitution system is required or preferred for acoustic reception.

Future development of high-resolution tactile systems may provide a substitute for vision. Very little is known about how age-related changes might influence information transmission through the skin, and even less is known about how pathological changes in skin or nerve affect functional sensation, orientation, and movement.

Age-related changes broaden the range of ergonomic variables that must be considered in developing new devices and appliances for use by older persons. If such design included the attributes of populations with the most common visual, hearing, tactile, and motor limitations, substantially expanded markets might emerge. These products would be of great benefit for home use and in health care settings. Such developments could effectively alter health care environments, treatment modalities, and living arrangements. Greater emphasis upon visual displays, acoustic signals and alarms, audibility levels, and tactile discriminability in home appliances, along with more effective communication systems and flexible transportation systems, could effectively prevent many of the barriers that transform impairment into disability. Despite major advancements, the fact still remains that most deaf older persons do not have access to the telephone.

REFERENCES

Bridges, J. A., & Bentler, R. A. (1998). Related hearing aid use to well-being among older adults. *The Hearing Journal, 51*(7), 39-51.

Cain, W., & Stevens, J. (1990). Missing ingredients: Aging and the discrimination of flavor. *Journal of Nutrition for the Elderly, 9*, 3-15.

Carmen, R. (1999). Sensorineural Insights. Part 1: Aging: It may never be too late. *Hearing Health, 15*(1), 21-24.

Chop, W. C., & Robnett, R. H. (1999). *Gerontology for the Health Care Professional.* Philadelphia: F.A. Davis.

Cox, R. & Alexander, G. (1995). The abbreviated profile of hearing aid benefit. *Ear & Hearing, 16* (2), 176-183.

DiGiovanna, A. G. (1994). *Human Aging.* New York: McGraw-Hill.

Ferrand, C. T., & Bloom, R. L. (1997). *Introduction to Organic and Neurogenic Disorders of Communication.* Needham Heights, MA: Allyn & Bacon.

Graaf, C., Polet, P., & Stavern, W. (1994). Sensory perception and pleasantness of food flavors in elderly subjects. *Journal of Gerontology, 49* (3), 93-99.

Hamdy, R. C. (1984). *Geriatric Medicine.* Philadelphia: Bailliere Tindall.

Hull, R. H. (1995). *Hearing in Aging.* San Diego: Singular Publishing Group, Inc.

Kart, C. S. (1997). *The Realities of Aging.* Boston: Allyn & Bacon.

Kart, C. S., Metress, E. K., & Metress, S. P. (1992). *Human Aging and Chronic Disease.* Boston: Jones and Bartlett.

Kricos, P. B., & Lesner, S. A. (1995). *Hearing Care for the Older Adult.* Philadelphia: W. B. Saunders Co.

Lesnoff-Caravaglia, G. (Ed.). (1988). *Aging in a Technological Society.* New York: Human Sciences Press.

Lesnoff-Caravaglia, G. (Ed.) (1987). *Handbook of Applied Gerontology.* New York: Human Sciences Press.

Lesnoff-Caravaglia, G. (Ed.). (1988). *International Journal of Technology and Aging, 1.*

Lord, S., Clark, R., & Webster, I. Postural stability and associated physiological factors in a population of aged persons. *Journal of Gerontology, 46* (3), M69-M76.

Oram, J. J. (1997). *Caring for the Fourth Age.* London: Armelle.

Sataloff, R. T., & Sataloff, J. (1993). *Hearing Loss.* New York: Marcel Dekker, Inc.

Shimon, D. A. (1992). *Coping With Hearing Loss and Hearing Aids.* San Diego: Singular Publishing Group, Inc.

Smith, R. (Ed.). (1997). *Aging Issue.* (Special Issue). *British Medical Journal, 315* (7115).

Spence, A. (1997). *Biology of Aging* (2nd ed.). Englewood Cliffs, NJ: Prentice-Hall.

U.S. Congress, Office of Technology Assessment. (1985). *Technology and Aging in America.* OTA-BA-265. Washington, DC: U.S. Government Printing Office.

Walter, J., & Soliah, L. (1995). Sweetener preference among non-institutionalized older adults. *Journal of Nutrition for the Elderly, 14*, 1-13.

Chapter 12

PSYCHOSOCIAL ISSUES

Biological changes experienced by older persons are either accommodated or exacerbated by the environment. The environment includes social, political, health care, and economic features, as well as the physical construct of the world in which they live.

The changing roles of older persons, and the presence of several family generations (which calls for a flexibility in role of the older person), are advents of the contemporary age. There is the factor of *role reversal*, in which adult children assume a parenting role toward aged parents. In addition, there is the increasing adoption of *role repetition* (resumption of the nurturant role for adult and elderly children, and for young grandchildren), as well as *role equivalence* whereby older persons by reason of age share the same social stereotyping with adult and aged children (i.e., mother, 98; daughter, 75) because of the general categorization of all persons over the age of 65 as "old."

Psychosocial issues play a significant role in the lives of older persons. This is particularly true in the case of women since women are predominant in the older population. As women grow older, their life experiences alter immeasurably.

The Older Woman

Women who are currently septuagenarians or older, probably have never engaged in gainful employment outside the home. This configuration will continue to change significantly as women of all ages increasingly enter the work force outside the home. In the past, women were completely reliant upon males for their maintenance, their standard of living, and their quality of life. Many of the cultural trends which continue today derive from such dependant status, such as the emphasis on female attractiveness to attract a husband to support her, the emphasis upon housekeeping skills or home management for women of all social classes, and the dominance of males as masters of the home because of their role as "bread-winners." Women continue to have difficulty in asserting their abilities and strengths in the world of work largely due to this historical role of females as cloistered and subordinate.

As a result, women still suffer from their lack of knowledge in the fields of finance and the mechanics of managing in the business world and its formalities. For the older woman, business dealings are hard to comprehend, and they rely principally on other males, relatives or professional persons, to assist them. The negative stereotyping of older females continues to foster the view of them as "helpless" in business matters. Unfortunately, some older women also accept this view of themselves. Such negative stereotyping of older men may appear but in milder form, if at all. Older women, however, have to combat this negative attitude, along with their unfamiliarity with the world of business.

The female role was to marry, to have children, to be a good mother and wife, and, if she carried all these duties out successfully, she probably had a place reserved for her in heaven. Women began to learn, however, that by the time they reached the age of 50 or 60, since they had married men who were older than themselves, they would very likely be left alone due to the death of the spouse. The status of being a couple was seriously eroded and disappeared as a crutch to support a maladaptive orientation toward life. The absence of the husband and the absence of a major buffer between oneself and the world, led to intense grief and major personal disorientation.

The social circle which had largely been determined by the husband's profession or occupation, found her less acceptable as a single person. The ties were based on work associations with a tolerance of the wife. Once the husband was gone, the wife was without social moorings. Most widows were far from "merry," and were for the most part lonely, uncertain individuals ill-equipped to handle the practical demands of daily life.

Increases in life expectancy have been mixed blessings for older women, particularly those who had seen their roles mirrored in social expectations. The longer they lived, the more superfluous they felt. They had raised their families, been good mothers and wives, and nursed the husbands in ill health until death. There was less and less opportunity to exercise traditional roles, and little guidance as to what new roles older women should adopt. Older women began to regard their lives as essentially lives of betrayal. They had conducted themselves according to societal expectations, and, once old and alone, they were abandoned by the very society they had thought to serve. They had been led to believe that if they did all of the expected things, there would be some sort of reward in the end. They did not expect to grow old alone. To grow old female was a role-less role. Depression and alcohol dependency faced many such women.

Also, in terms of assistance in old age, many older women had to look to social and health service agencies. The death of the spouse and the distance separating her from offspring led to lives of isolation.

Societal expectations for women were biological in nature. They were expected to marry, to have children, to care for ailing relatives, to nurse their husbands and to bury them. The role was essentially a nurturing one. Once such duties were accomplished, society forgot about them. The children grew up, married and left home; the husband became ill, was nursed by her and died. His funeral was, in fact, her social death.

In more recent years, such vacancies and changes in the family have meant increased freedom for the older woman. Older women have returned to academic and training institutions for preparation to enter new or interrupted careers. The "empty nest" rather than encouraging depression, provided a sense of freedom women had not experienced since marriage.

Unfortunately, not all women were so well equipped to meet the new challenges of life. Many had fragmented educational experiences, work histories that were full of gaps of years due to childbearing and rearing, checkered employment patterns, and unequal contributions to pension and insurance plans.

For many years the only occupations open to women were strictly aligned to their nurturing roles. She could become a teacher, nurse, or possibly a social worker. She was viewed as most capable in caring for children or in a form of nurturing role. Teachers colleges were often established in rural settings so that the future teacher would remain clear of worldly distractions and would see her vocation something similar to that of a nun. In fact, for many years teachers were expected to remain single, and upon marriage, had to leave the classroom. This was not true of male teachers.

The reproductive role has become something of an anachronism since the advent of contraceptives. Women now live more years in a state of non-procreation, than as sexually productive. Women who have lived to advanced ages have also provided society with examples of active, independent women. It is not necessary to look to famous figures such as Grandma Moses, but to simply look next door to see a woman in her eighties or nineties living alone and functioning very well.

Attitudes of health care personnel have limited the treatments accessible to older women, and the absence of sufficient research has seriously circumscribed the knowledge of women's health issues.

Independence, Dependence, and Disability

The shifting age structure of society has caused changes in the prevalence and composition of disability. The shift toward gradually decreasing functional abilities as a result of age or chronic illness is producing a new population of individuals who would benefit from assistance, but who might be classified as "disabled" in the traditional sense. By the year 2020, 22 million persons will be aged 75 or older.

The shift in demography also suggests a smaller working-age labor force and hence fewer workers to care for disabled persons. Such an increase among octogenarians, nonagenarians and centenarians implies a greater burden to existing health care providers. While some within this burgeoning aging population may well enjoy better health than do people in the same age bracket today, many will require increased health services. Also, since the size of the population is becoming greater, this will also add to the strain upon the health care system. Such demand may be partly met by technology working in concert with human caregivers to augment human caregiving capabilities.

Over the past several decades the growth of the elderly population has been an unprecedented phenomenon; however, during this time, knowledge about aging has increased significantly. Also during this time, many technological advances have been achieved. It is the coming together of these three occurrences—the growth in the aging population, increased knowledge about aging, and current technological advances as well as expected future advances, that contribute to what might well be a unique historical period.

The increased life expectancy in the population contains both negative and positive features. Although people are living longer, they will be surviving into ages wherein the prevalence of chronic and debilitating conditions, in addition to the acute diseases many elderly experience, have severe implications for quality of life and maintenance of independence in old age.

Old age does not necessarily mean a state of disability and dependency, because many older people are able to live independent and relatively healthy lives even into advanced old age. Although new advances in medicine have led to the prevention and control of many diseases, there remains considerable disability among the aging population.

Eight percent or more of persons over the age of 65 have at least one identifiable chronic disease or condition. The most common conditions are arthritis, impaired hearing or vision, diabetes, chronic heart disease, and some degree of mental impairment. These conditions often lead to the inability to perform the activities of daily living. Limitations in activities of daily living (ADL) (walking, bathing, dressing, eating, getting in and out of bed, and toileting) are an important indicator of loss of independence in the elderly and reflect the impact of major chronic diseases on the functioning of the older person.

If these age-specific rates of disability continue into the next century, by the year 2040, for every 100 older persons, 13 will have significant disability, a 36 percent increase that results simply from the change in age distribution of those 65 and over. It is estimated that this will result in 8.6 million older disabled persons.

Robotic Technologies

Robotic technologies can be developed that can assist in personal care tasks and activities of daily living, such as cooking and feeding, grooming, and retrieval and placement of items (fetch and carry tasks); recreational tasks such as board games and painting; vocationally related tasks such as opening file drawers, extracting files, and inserting disks into computers.

Robotic technologies for caregivers can replace odious, routine, demeaning, or boring tasks and allow the health care provider the opportunity to deliver care that humans can uniquely provide. In this way, the robotic technology is potentially augmenting their quality caregiving by reducing some of its more burdensome aspects. Fetch-and-carry tasks, lifting and transferring, vital-signs monitoring, feeding, and bowel and bladder care are all tasks in which technology can significantly assist.

Insufficient information is available with respect to ergonomics, strength, neuromuscular, biomechanical, and perceptual variables of either disabled or older populations. An additional complication derives from the difficulty associated with the stigma "disabled" or "handicapped." Many individuals, especially older persons, prefer not to think of themselves as disabled or handicapped because they have some gradual loss in functional capabilities. Few persons view themselves as "visually handicapped" because they wear glasses or contact lenses. Such interventions, however, are assistive devices that reduce the functional limitations resulting from impaired eyesight.

Applications for Robotic Technology

There are robots at work indirectly in the human service sectors of research and diagnostic laboratories. Robots are extensively used to perform routine laboratory tasks from sample preparation to radioimmunoassays. Such application of robots is particularly useful in handling agents associated with communicable diseases such as tuberculosis, AIDS, or other substances dangerous to humans.

The range of applications for robotic technology in health and social services will vary according to their use in particular environments. Like all machines, their specific use will determine the type and level of design. Tasks amenable to robotic technology include housekeeping, ambulation, transfer-lift-transport of patients, physical therapy, depuddler (cleaning up of urine spills), surveillance (wandering patients), physician assistant, nurse assistant, patient assistant, vital-signs monitoring, and mental stimulation.

Settings in which such technological interventions would be appropriate include emergency/urgent care units, hospitals, skilled-nursing facilities, and residential, in-home and ambulatory sites. Major questions concerning safety, effectiveness, reliability, cost savings, and serviceability must be addressed.

Automated Guided Vehicle Systems (AGVS) technology is already beginning to be employed in institutional health care environments to transport meals, drinks, and personal items to patients. Such a mobile robotic device could also move from patient to patient and collect vital signs data, and, with two-way communication, provide a link with the centralized nursing station.

Robotic technology holds the possibility for playing a role in both patient therapy and therapist training. The human therapist has a finite amount of energy, whereas robotic technologies can continue providing therapy indefinitely. There is also a reduced risk of back injuries to the therapist, and reduced insurance costs to the facility.

Robots may come in many forms and sizes, according to their precise function. They could range from the efficient, machinelike devices to those with more human-like attributes. The robot could present characteristics that give it "personality" through voice, appearance, and movement.

Mobility and Technological Advances

The technological advances that have achieved a significant extension of the duration of life have also resulted in achieving improvement in the quality of life. Specifically, these advances have dramatically enhanced the ability to be mobile. Mobility that is conducive to walking, as well as small-muscle coordination, is essential to activities of daily living.

Surgical technology can improve eyesight, retard joint degeneration, and reduce deafness. Pharmaceutical technology has improved the medications for the maintenance of chronic conditions and the elimination of acute ones. Advances in science, technology and medicine have allowed for research into cellular and molecular behavior, which is resulting in the retarding of aging and in facilitating the maintenance of health. In many ways, yet to be devised, technology is the stimulus for maintaining youthful, spontaneous, and efficient behaviors. Technology has been responsible for the slowing of the aging process and for improving the general quality of life.

As technology produces assistive devices with greater accuracy and sensitivity, it works inherently to improve healthful behaviors. Technology reduces physical difficulties, but it needs to concomitantly foster the development of the person who emerges as a result of the integration of the person and the technology. The person created by such integration should emerge as one more unique and more personally satisfying than was the previous self. Thus technology can serve as a new evolutionary force that does not simply retard aging, but that can lead to undeveloped and unsuspected levels of human experiencing as people grow old. This approach recognizes the encroachments of biological aging, but views such changes as challenges, not as detriments to growth and development. Technology, thus, can help foster new developmental tasks for the aged populations.

Social Theories of Aging

The theories that have long been promulgated as to how older persons deal with long life have provided more questions and criticisms than helpful answers. The disengagement theory long held that older persons willingly removed themselves from society. They withdrew from social participation and prepared for their own demise.

The theory that probably best explains people's attitudes toward aging is the continuity theory. This simply states that persons wish to continue in their pursuits and activities which have always made their lives meaningful.

Elder Abuse and Victimization

The increase in the older population has also increased the awareness of older persons as targets for criminal activity and abuse by caregivers in both the familial and institutional setting. Elder abuse has grown as a social problem, and many states now have mandatory reporting laws similar to that in child abuse.

The greater numbers of older persons means that there is a concomitant increase in the number and types of health and social problems that are conducive to acts of violence against older persons. Dependency upon caregivers and caregivers who are dependant upon older persons provide a scenario fraught with economic, health, and interpersonal problems. Abuse can be physical, emotional or psychological. The hidden nature of such abuse and the reluctance of older persons to admit to being victims at the hands of relatives helps perpetrate this problem. Spousal abuse can also continue into old age.

Economic factors, lack of personal self-esteem, health problems, and economic concerns also contribute to conditions of helplessness and hopelessness which increasingly lead to the victimization of older persons. Such abusive patterns may reflect familial discord, burn out on the part of caregivers, revengeful behaviors, substance abuse on the part of the older person or the caregiver, or society's condoning violent behavior.

Older persons are also increasingly victims of criminal behavior. Their established routines and use of public transportation makes them particularly vulnerable. The increase of sensory loss makes older persons more likely to be targets for criminal actions.

The Diogenes Syndrome

The Diogenes Syndrome is a form of extreme self-neglect, poorly understood, which is a form of self-abuse. It is named after the Greek philosopher who reputedly lived his life in a tub surrounded by squalor. He also walked in daylight hours through the streets of Athens in Greece carrying a lighted lantern, looking for an honest man.

This syndrome appears to have linkages to losses of a significant other, resulting in total distrust. The condition is found among the poor and the wealthy, and cuts across socioeconomic lines. It can be described as a form of self burial. Some recluses may also harbor animals such as cats or dogs in large numbers, while others have rooms full of collections of old newspapers, magazines, refuse.

Such older persons reject any services, and usually come to the attention of health care providers through the emergency services.

General Characteristics of Illness in Old Age

One of the bigger problems of illness in old age is that in many ways it appears as a social problem rather than an illness. For example, if a woman aged 80 years of age can no longer do her shopping, her family or friends usually contact a social service agency and arrange for a homemaker to do the shopping. Meanwhile, the prime cause of why she cannot shop is ignored. The next stage may be difficulty getting upstairs to bed and possibly also to the bathroom. The reaction is to bring the bed downstairs and to arrange for a commode to be located nearby. Eventually, a downstairs existence deteriorates into a one-room existence. Each deterioration is met with increased assistance from family members or social services offering a variety of help. In this way, remedial medical problems are often overlooked and not dealt with until it is too late.

Weight loss and poor appetite are frequently attributed to old age, even if the older person routinely goes to see his or her doctor. Treatable cancers, for example, can be missed for a period of months or even years.

Traditionally, the patient goes to the doctor with a specific complaint of pain or a swelling, but this model of presentation in the elderly is rare. They often accept gradual slowing down due to arthritis, breathlessness, or tiredness as due to old age. As a result, they present a level of frailty and disability which passes unnoticed by them and by their families. Consequently, it is not brought to the attention of the physician. Acceptance of aging is an important part of survival, but it does lead to the overlooking of problems such as sight or hearing loss and dental deterioration.

Disability and Dependence

The frustration of disability in old age is the frequent reliance on someone else for care even when mentally the individual may be very alert. Such caregivers, particularly aged children or spouses, may also be at risk related to their own problems of coping, disease, or stress.

The problems of old age are not mental or social, but the result of the natural processes of aging. Some characteristics of disease in old age include: multiple illness; acute onset and rapid death; insidious onset and silent existence; impaired homeostatic mechanisms; impaired drug tolerance; confusional states; impaired immune function; and secondary consequences of immobility—incontinence or pressure sores.

Long-Term Care

Long-term care for the elderly includes a variety of health and social services provided for individuals who need assistance because of physical or mental disability. Technologies appropriate for addressing those needs and improving services and service delivery include: assessment technologies to identify functional impairments and facilitate matching of the individual with long-term care services; technologies to maintain or increase independent functioning, including assistive devices and rehabilitation services; technologies to assist formal and informal caregivers; and service delivery systems to improve access to appropriate long-term care.

Although there is no single accepted definition of long-term care, it is generally agreed that the goal of long-term care is to maintain or improve the ability of the individual to function as independently as possible and that services will be needed over a prolonged period, even if they are only needed intermittently. Medical care is seen as an essential component of long-term care, but a variety of other services are also considered important.

Long-term care is generally concerned with functional impairments, such as limitations in the individual's ability to move around independently; to feed, dress, or bathe him or herself; or to perform housekeeping functions such as shopping, cooking, or cleaning. While acute care is most often directed toward treating or curing disease, long-term care is generally directed toward compensating for functional impairment and maintaining or improving the functional capacity of the individual.

Approximately one and a half million elderly are residents in nursing homes at any one time. Approximately another half million are residents of board and care facilities, many elderly persons are receiving one or more long-term care services in their homes or communities. Adult day care facilities, hospice programs, and congregate housing facilities also provide long-term care services in some communities.

The need for formal long-term care services is expected to increase dramatically in the future as a result of rapid growth in the number of elderly individuals in the population. Over the past half century, advances in public sanitation, hygiene, and medical care have lowered mortality from infectious diseases, and individuals who might have died earlier of these causes now live long enough to develop functional impairments related to chronic diseases. Medical treatment has also lowered mortality from heart attacks, strokes, and some cancers, but there is currently no evidence that the onset of chronic disease and functional impairment has been postponed.

Home Health Care

Health care services provided in the home include medical, social, and supportive services designed to maintain the individual in the community and to compensate for impaired functioning. Even with the experience of two or more chronic diseases, many older persons are capable of remaining in the community with the assistance of home health care.

Most older persons prefer to live in their own homes for as long as possible. The home is a familiar environment, and the person has learned over a number of years how to negotiate this environment to meet his or her specific needs. The home may even take on a prosthetic nature. For most persons, moving to a new environment can be very disorienting and can lead to mental or physical deterioration. A familiar environment promotes self-esteem and independence, a sense of identity, protection, and comfort. Persons who suffer from some mental confusion can still manage in a familiar environment. People removed from a familiar environment can suffer what has been termed the "relocation effect" which can result, not only in compromising the person's health, but possibly even death.

Assistance from health and social service agencies and family members are important factors in maintaining the independence of the older and more frail population. Programs such as Meals on Wheels which deliver meals to the home, respite care, chore services, and friendly visitors all contribute to the maintenance of the older person's independence and well-being.

Personal Identity

Many of the changes older persons experience are both internal and external. Since external changes are most obvious to the person, physical changes may be viewed with alarm. Some older persons have difficulty in accepting their changed appearance and their altered level of functioning. Women are particularly concerned over physical attractiveness, while men are concerned over changes in body size, loss of muscle, and fear of impotence.

The shortened stature of older persons is due to changes in the vertebral column or might be due to osteoporosis. Diseases such as osteoporosis have their onset in early mid-life and a lifetime habit of limiting the amount of dairy products results in ingesting smaller amounts of calcium which, in turn, can result in osteoporosis. Older persons also have a tendency to stoop which may be the result of years of poor posture.

Proper posture is beneficial to internal organs and allows the respiratory system to function at a higher level. Exercise programs to teach older persons correct posture need to be instituted. Learning to balance the body and learning to walk correctly is a preventive measure that would benefit many older persons. Information on proper foot attire and the development of appropriate footwear is a neglected area in the health care of older adults.

Exercise, diet control to prevent obesity, and constant movement to offset muscle rigidity are important aspects of mobility. Disuse of the body results in an inability to achieve proper movement. The numbers of persons in nursing homes who spend their lives bedfast locked in a fetal position are good examples of stationery lives. Unfortunately, the blind and the deaf too often end their lives in this state.

Stressful Events

Life events such as experiencing the death of a spouse or close relative can result in psychological as well as physical responses. The reaction to grief varies among individuals, but it is commonly accepted that it takes the average person about a year to recover from a death.

Amputation of a limb is another traumatic loss. As people live longer and more persons are afflicted with diabetes mellitus, the rate of amputation among older persons has increased. Some people elect to die rather than to lose a limb.

Surgery in old age, unless the person is adequately prepared, can be a stressful event. Recovery from surgery for some persons proceeds at a rather slow pace, and depression can result.

In most animal species, animals do not live long beyond the period of reproduction. Women who experience menopause from the ages of 45 to 55 on the average, live on for a number of years. This life beyond reproduction has provided freedom for women, but, also, for some, anxiety. There are also biological changes that come into play following the onset of menopause.

Suicide

Suicide, as a form of death, has long been regarded as a societal taboo. Such avoidance of the subject of suicide has been true of health care professionals, and the general public alike. Throughout history, suicide has been regarded as a sin or a crime, or both. It is a sin, in part, in that one does kill oneself, and this is considered by many as an act contrary to religious tenets. Furthermore, there is no opportunity for a last confession, the last rites, which form part of the sacraments at death in some religious groups. Suicide is a crime because it is contrary to the cultural order of some societies. Such evaluations of suicide, however, were formulated when life expectancy did not exceed 50 years.

As in other age groups, clues to older suicides are both obvious and masked. Nonetheless, even very obvious clues are frequently not detected by health care personnel or caretakers, simply because changes in behavior of older persons are not closely monitored, or when different, are ascribed to negative aspects of aging, such as withdrawal.

Some clues include putting one's affairs in order or deliberately exposing oneself to danger. Causes may stem from loss of any of the special senses, the prospect of being institutionalized, the unexpected experience of economic difficulties, dramatic changes in self-image (amputation), the death of a spouse, or a feeling of uselessness and of being a burden on one's family.

The perspective on suicide varies between different age groups. Younger persons may view suicide as a form of escape; older persons who decide to commit suicide mean to die. The motives for younger persons may include a disappointing love affair, failed exams, loss of job, or depression. The motives for older persons include the loss of meaningful relationships through death, loss of home, insurmountable practical problems, chronic pain or illness, or a combination of several irreversible factors. Older persons do not usually have a history of prior attempts, and their suicide is the result of a long planning process.

The greatest fear of suicidal older persons is that they may not be successful. An unsuccessful suicide attempt can result in greater debilitation and worsened conditions. The method to be employed and the timing has to be carefully selected. Furthermore, older persons often do not have the strength or capability to carry out a suicide plan and must resort to life-threatening behaviors such as medical non-compliance and refusal of nourishment. Some seek to enlist the help of a caregiver.

Life-Sustaining Technologies

Modern science has brought about dramatic changes in medical care and now gives people considerable power to alter both the quality and length of human life. It has also raised difficult questions with respect to individual rights, the processes of living and dying, and the proper distribution of technological resources.

In decisionmaking about life-sustaining technologies, distinctions are sometimes made between withholding versus withdrawing treatment, direct versus indirect effects of actions, letting die and killing, and ordinary and extraordinary means of treatment. In addition to the ethical distinctions involved in treating individual patients, there are significant ethical issues associated with the way in which life-sustaining technologies are allocated, shared or distributed. The use of life-sustaining technologies for older persons are closely related to the economics of their use.

As equipment and procedures have been refined and experiences accumulated, the necessary personnel, facilities, and reimbursement have expanded, and the clinical criteria guiding use have been broadened. The types of patients who become candidates for life-sustaining treatments have changed, and their numbers have increased sharply. Many of these patients are older individuals. What were once considered extraordinary measures have become commonplace, as more constantly powerful technologies emerge.

Technologies that support or replace the functioning of a vital organ are capable of saving and sustaining life, and sometimes, capable of restoring health and independence. It is never clear, however, if a particular life-sustaining technology will sustain the life of a particular patient or, if it does, for how long. The quality of the life that is sustained may be even harder to predict. An important factor that further complicates matters is that many patients with life-threatening conditions are not able to understand their treatment options or to express preferences regarding them.

At any one time, many thousands of elderly persons are receiving life-sustaining interventions. The vast majority of cases go unnoticed except by the patients, family members, and others directly involved in making and living with difficult treatment decisions.

Life-sustaining technologies are drugs, medical devices, or procedures that can keep individuals alive who would otherwise die within a foreseeable, but usually uncertain, time period.

Global Aging

The demography of aging is now being defined in terms of two different dimensions: one dealing with what might be called the demography of population aging and the second dealing with the demography of the aged population. There is extensive population aging on a global basis. These developments are occurring, of course, at different times in various regions of the world. It is important to pay attention not only to the numbers of older people, but also the proportions of older people in total populations. It is important to check sex distribution as well as dependency ratios–ratios of older persons to younger persons and older persons to the working aged population. These are imbedded aspects of the process of population aging that have important and often direct implications on policy issues concerned with the allocation of resources and transfers of resources between generations.

It often comes as a surprise that not only is the general population aging, but that particular subgroups within this population continue to age as well. Such groups include the mentally ill, the developmentally disabled, persons with a variety of physical handicaps, those who suffer from chronic illnesses, along with prison inmates. The prison population includes persons who have grown old in prison, as well as those who are imprisoned late in life. Since all these older groups eventually present with the problems of senescence and chronic illness, they represent significant and problematic groups within the aging population.

There has been growing attention given to the aging of the prison population in the United States, and to the increase in its numbers in recent years. The appropriateness of separating older inmates from younger inmates for reasons of safety, and the provision of appropriate housing and health care are major issues. One consequence has been the taxing of health care expenditures; providing for prisoners who are reaching advanced ages with deteriorating health has proven very costly.

Not only is the total population aging, but there is, in addition, the aging of the aged population. This growth has important implications in terms of gender balance in that a high proportion of the octogenarians and nonagenarians are females. This raises specific issues relating to widowhood and other needs of older women, both social and health-related, deriving from their greater longevity compared to men.

A great deal of attention has been paid to the baby-boomers who will reach the older ages in the second decade of the new millennium and what their increased presence will mean. This is a concern not only of more developed countries, but also for developing countries, which experienced extremely high fertility rates following World War II. The climate in which aging will be experienced in the future will be determined, not only by economic factors, but, also, by the understanding that is brought to the nature of aging.

REFERENCES

Barber, H. (1996). Preoperative and postoperative care of the elderly women. *Clinical Obstetrics and Gynecology, 39* (4), 902-905.

Brooks, L., Wertsch, J., et. al. (1994). Use of devices for mobility by the elderly. *Wisconsin Medical Journal,* 16-20.

Butler, R. N., & Body, J.A. (Ed.). (1995). *Delaying the Onset of Late-Life Dysfunction.* New York: Springer.

Crabtree, J., & Caron-Parker, L. Long-term care of the aged: Ethical dilemmas and solutions. *The American Journal of Occupational Therapy, 45,* 607-612.

Davis, M. A., Moritz, D., Neuhaus, J., et.al. (1997). Living arrangements, changes in living arrangements, and survival among community dwelling older adults. *American Journal of Public Health, 87* (3), 210-216.

Fernie, G. (1994). Technology to assist elderly people's safe mobility. *Experimental Aging Research, 20,* 219-228.

Fleming, B. E., & Pendergast, D. (1993). Physical condition, activity pattern, and environment as factors in falls by adult care facility residents. *Archives of Physical Medicine Rehabilitation, 74,* 627-630.

Harris, R. (Ed.). (1983). *Medical devices and instrumentation for the elderly.* Arlington, VA: Association for the Advancement of Medical Instrumentation.

Hobson, D. (1993). Technology for seniors' living environment: Directions for product development. *Experimental Aging Research, 20,* 291-301.

Lesnoff-Caravaglia, G. (Ed.). (1987). *Aging in a Technological Society.* New York: Human Sciences Press.

Lesnoff-Caravaglia, G. (Ed.). (1988). *Handbook of Applied Gerontology.* New York: Human Sciences Press.

Oram, J.J. (1997). *Caring for the Fourth Age.* London, UK: Armelle Press.

Parker, M., & Thorslund, M. (1990). The use of technical aids among community based elderly. *American Journal of Occupational Therapy, 45,* 712-717.

Rapp, K., & Rapp, M.P. (1993). Challenges to quality care in Texas nursing facilities. *Texas Medicine, 89* (10), 62-66.

Technology Application and the Elderly. (1980). (Report). Glastonbury, CT: The Futures Group.

U.S. Congress, Office of Technology Assessment. (1987). *Life-sustaining technologies and the elderly.* OTA-BA-306. Washington, DC: U.S. Government Printing Office.

U.S. Congress, Office of Technology Assessment. (1985). *Technology and aging in America.* Washington, DC: U.S. Government Printing Office.

Ware, C., (Ed.). (1993). *Strategies for collaboration between architects and occupational therapists.* Washington, DC: Aging Design Research Program.

BIBLIOGRAPHY

Allen, G., & Derose, J. (1997). Pulmonary nodule resection during lung volume reduction surgery. *AORN Journal, 66* (5), 808-818.

Andrews, G. R. (Ed). (1998). Aging beyond 2000: One world one future. *Australian Journal on Ageing, 17* (1), Supplement.

Arnow, W., & Tresch, D. (1997). Treatment of congestive heart failure in older persons. *JAGS,45* (10), 1252-1257.

Barber, H. (1996). Preoperative and postoperative care of the elderly women. *Clinical Obstetrics and Gynecology, 39* (4), 902-905.

Bengtson, V. L., & Schaie, K. W. (1999). *Handbook of Theories of Aging.* New York: Springer.

Blazer, D. (1997). *Emotional Problems in Later Life* (2nd ed). New York: Springer.

Bloom, B. (1990). Medical management and managing medical care: The dilemma of evaluating new technology. *American Heart Journal, 199* (3), 754-761.

Boling, P. (1997). *The Physicians's Role in Home Health Care.* New York: Springer.

Brooks, L., Wertsch, J., et al. (1994). Use of devices for mobility by the elderly. *Wisconsin Medical Journal,* 16-20.

Butler, R. N., & Brody, J. A., (Eds.). (1995). *Delaying the Onset of Late-Life Dysfunction.* New York: Springer.

Cain, W., & Stevens, J. (1990). Missing ingredients: Aging and the discrimination of flavor. *Journal of Nutrition for the Elderly, 9,* 3-15.

Chandra, R. (1995). Nutrition and immunity in the elderly: Clinical significance. *Nutrition Review, 53* (4), s80-s85.

Chop, W. C., & Robnett, R. H. (1999). *Gerontology for the Health Care Professional.* Philadelphia: F.A. Davis.

Coleman, P.G. (1999). Creating a life story: The task of reconciliation. *The Gerontologist, 39* (2), 133-139.

Colt, H., Ries, A., et al. (1997). Analysis of chronic obstructive pulmonary disease referrals for lung volume reduction surgery. *Journal of Cardiopulmonary Rehabilitation, 17,* 248-252.

Coombs, F. (1994). Engineering technology in rehabilitation of older adults. *Experimental Aging Research, 20,* 201-209.

Crabtree, J., & Caron-Parker, L. Long-term care of the aged: Ethical dilemmas and solutions. *The American Journal of Occupational Therapy, 45,* 607-612.

Danenberg, H. D., & Ben-Yuhuda, A. et. al. (1997). Dehydroepiandrosterone treatment is not beneficial to the immune response to influenza in elderly subjects. *Journal of Clinical Endocrinology & Metabolism, 82,* 2911-4.

DiGiovanna, A. G. (1994). *Human Aging.* New York: McGraw-Hill.

Englehardt, K.G. (1989). Health and human service robotics: Multi-dimensional perspectives. *International Journal of Technology and Aging, 2* (1), 6-41.

Evers, M., Townsend, C., & Thompson, J. (1994). Organ physiology of aging. *Surgical Clinics of North America, 74* (1), 23-39.

Fernie, G. (1994). Technology to assist elderly people's safe mobility. *Experimental Aging Research, 20,* 219-228.

Fleming, B.E., & Pendergast, D. (1993). Physical condition, activity pattern, and environment as factors in falls by adult care facility residents. *Archives of Physical Medicine Rehabilitation, 74,* 627-630.

Freedman, A., Hahn, G., & Love, N. (1996). Follow-up therapy for prostate cancer. *Postgraduate Medicine, 100* (3), 125-134.

Garrett, T. M., Baillie, H. W., & Garrett, R. M. (1993). *Health Care Ethics* (2nd ed.). Englewood Cliffs, NJ: Prentice Hall.

Gitlin, L., Levine, R. & Geiger, C. (1993). Adaptive device use by older adults with mixed disabilities. *Archives of Physical Medicine Rehabilitation, 73,* 149-152.

Godschalk, M., Sison, A., & Mulligan, T. (1997). Management of erectile dysfunction by the geriatrician. *JAGS, 45* (10), 1240-1246.

Goldenberg, K., & Faryna, A. (Eds.). (1990). *Geriatric Medicine for the House Officer.* Baltimore: Williams and Wilkins.

Graaf, C., Polet, P., & Staveren, W. (1994). Sensory perception and pleasantness of food flavors in elderly subjects. *Journal of Gerontology, 49* (3), 93-99.

Hamdy, R. C. (1984). *Geriatric Medicine.* Philadelphia: Bailliere Tindall.

Hampton, J. K., Craven, R. F., & Heitkemper, M. M. (1997). *The Biology of Human Aging* (2nd ed.). Dubuque, IA: Wm. C. Brown.

Harris, R. (Ed.). (1983). *Medical devices and instrumentation for the elderly.* Arlington, VA: Association for the Advancement of Medical Instrumentation.

Haub, M.R. (1994). Elderly patients, caregivers, and physicians: Theory and research on health care triads. *Journal of Health and Social Behavior, 35,* 1-12.

Hobson, D. (1993). Technology for senior's living environment: Directions for product development. *Experimental Aging Research, 20,* 291-301.

Howell, S. (1994). The potential environment: Home, technology and future aging. *Experimental Aging Research, 20,* 285-290.

Janicki, M. P., & Dalton, A. J. (1998). *Dementia, Aging, and Intellectual Disabilities.* Philadelphia: Brunner/Mazel.

Kart, C. S. (1997). *The Realities of Aging.* Boston: Allyn & Bacon.

Kart, C. S., Metress, E. K., & Metress, S. P. (1992). *Human Aging and Chronic Disease.* Boston: Jones and Bartlett.

Kaye, L.W., & Davitt, J. K. (1999). *Current Practice in High-Tech Home Care.* New York: Springer.

Klerk, M., Huijsman, R., & McDonnell, J. (1997). The use of technical aids by elderly persons in the Netherlands: An application of the Andersen and Newman model. *The Gerontologist, 37* (3), 365-373.

Lesnoff-Caravaglia, G. (Ed.). (1984). *The World of the Older Woman.* New York: Human Sciences Press.

Lesnoff-Caravaglia, G. (Ed.). (1987). *Handbook of Applied Gerontology*. New York: Human Sciences Press.

Lesnoff-Caravaglia, G. (Ed.). (1988). *Aging in a Technological Society*. New York: Human Sciences Press.

Lesnoff-Caravaglia, G. (Ed.). (1988). *International Journal of Technology and Aging, 1* (1).

Lesnoff-Caravaglia, G. (Ed.). (1988). *International Journal of Technology and Aging, 1* (2).

Lesnoff-Caravaglia, G. (Ed.). (1989). *International Journal of Technology and Aging, 2* (1).

Lesnoff-Caravaglia, G. (Ed.). (1989). *International Journal of Technology and Aging, 2* (2).

Lesnoff-Caravaglia, G. (Ed.). (1990). *International Journal of Technology and Aging, 3* (1).

Lesnoff-Caravaglia, G. (Ed.). (1990). *International Journal of Technology and Aging, 3* (2).

Lesnoff-Caravaglia, G. (Ed.). (1991). *International Journal of Technology and Aging, 4* (1).

Lesnoff-Caravaglia, G. (Ed.). (1991). *International Journal of Technology and Aging, 4* (2).

Lesnoff-Caravaglia, G. (Ed.). (1992). *International Journal of Technology and Aging, 5* (1).

Lesnoff-Caravaglia, G. (Ed.). (1992). *International Journal of Technology and Aging 5* (2).

Lesnoff-Caravaglia, G., & Klys, M. (1987). An alternative paradigm for the study of aging. *Geriatrics, 35* (4), 366-368.

Lesnoff-Caravaglia, G., & Klys, M. (1987). Lifestyle and longevity. In G. Lesnoff-Caravaglia (Ed.). *Realistic Expectations for Long Life* (pp. 35-48). New York: Human Sciences Press.

Mann, W.C., Hurren, D., & Tomita, M. (1995). Assistive devices used by home-based elderly persons with arthritis. *The American Journal of Occupational Therapy, 49* (8), 810-819.

McConnel, E., & Murphy, E. (1990). Nurses' use of technology; An international concern. *International Nursing Review, 37* (5), 329-331.

Miller, K. (1996). Hormone replacement therapy in the elderly. *Clinical Obstetrics and Gynecology, 39* (4), 912-932.

Miller, L.D., Allen, S.M., et al. (1992). Videothoracoscopic wedge excision of the lung. *The Society of Thoracic Surgeons, 79* (9), 572-78.

Mumford, L. (1963). *Technics and Civilization*. New York: Harcourt, Brace & World.

Oram, J. J. (1997). *Caring for the Fourth Age*. London: Armelle.

Parker, M., & Thorslund, M. (1990). The use of technical aids among community based elderly. *American Journal of Occupational Therapy, 45*, 712-717.

Perler, B. (1994). Vascular disease in the elderly patient. *Surgical Clinics of North America, 74* (1), 199-216.

Quivey, M. (1990). Advanced medical technology: Finding the answers. *International Nursing Review, 37* (5), 329-331.

Rapp, K., Y Rapp, M.P. (1993). Challenges to quality care in Texas nursing facilities. *Texas Medicine, 89* (10), 62-66.

Robots revolutionize material transport at hospitals. (1999, March). RN, 62(3), 30.

Ross, I. K. (1995). *Aging of Cells, Humans & Societies*. Dubuque, IA: Wm. C. Brown Publishers.

Rowe, J. W., & Kahn, R. (1998). *Successful Aging*. New York: Pantheon.

Schulz, R., & Salthouse, T. (Eds.). (1995). *Adult Development and Aging* (3rd ed.). Upper Saddle River, NJ: Prentice-Hall.

Schneider, E. L., & Rose, J.W. (Eds.). (1990). *Handbook of the Biology of Aging* (3rd ed.). New York: Academic Press.

Smith, E. (Ed.). (1997). Aging Issue (special issue). *British Medical Journal, 315* (7115).

Spence, D.A. (1995). *Biology of Human Aging* (2nd ed.). Englewood Cliffs, NJ: Prentice-Hall.

Stolley, J. & Buckwalter, K. (1991). Iatrogenesis in the elderly. *Journal of Gerontological Nursing, 17* (9), 30-34.

Sunderkotter, C., Kalden, H., & Luger, T. (1997). Aging and the kin immune system. *ARCH Dermatology, 133*, 1256-1261.

Tallis, R., Fillit, H., & Brocklehurst, J. C. (Eds.). (1998). *Brocklehurst's Textbook of Geriatric Medicine and Gerontology* (5th ed.). London: Churchill Livingstone.

Taub, M., Begas, A. & Love, N. (1996). Advanced prostate cancer. *Postgraduate Medicine, 100* (3), 125-134.

U.S. Congress, Office of Technology Assessment. (1987). *Life-sustaining technologies and the elderly.* OTA-BA-306. Washington, DC: U.S. Government Printing Office.

U.S. Congress, Office of Technology Assessment. (1985). *Technology and aging in America.* OTA-BA-265. Washington, DC: U.S. Government Printing Office.

Utell, M., & Samet, J. (1990). Environmentally mediated disorders of the respiratory tract. *Medical Clinics of North America, 74* (2), 291-306.

Walter, J., & Soliah, L. (1995). Sweetener preference among non-institutionalized older adults. *Journal of Nutrition for the Elderly, 14*, 1-13.

Webster's New Collegiate Dictionary. (1989). Springfield, MA: Merriam-Webster.

Weiner, K. K., Long, R., Hughes, M., Chandler, J., et.al. (1993). When older adults face the chair-rise challenge. *JAGS, 41*, 6-10.

Weinstock, M. (1997). Death from skin cancer among the elderly. *ARCH Dermatology, 133*, 1207-1209.

Weksler, M. (1995). Immune senescence: Deficiency or dysregulation. *Nutrition Review, 53* (4), s3-s7.

Wick, G., & Grubeck-Loebenstein, B. (1997). The aging immune system: Primary and secondary alterations of immune reactivity in the elderly. *Experimental Gerontology, 32* (4), 401-413.

Winger, J., & Hornick, T. (1996). Age-associated changes in the endocrine system. *Nursing Clinics of North America, 31* (4), 827-844.

Zarit, S. H., & Zarit, J. M. (1998). *Mental Disorders in Older Adults.* New York: Guilford Publications.

INDEX